Powerful, heart-breaking and breathtaking. Benjamin draws you in and keeps you there. It's one thing to talk about hope, it's another to feel it! If you are suffering from any loss, this is the book for you. I highly recommend it.
~ Angie Cartwright, *Founder of National Grief Awareness Day*

Benjamin Allen's book, *Out of the Ashes*, is a must for anyone experiencing loss. I know this book would have benefited me years ago during my own journey with loss. The loss of the kind of life I would have with my daughter and the loss of my ten-year marriage. Thank you, Benjamin, for sharing your story and for investing so much time to share it in such a meaningful way.
~ Camilla Downs, *Author of "D is for Different - One Woman's Journey to Acceptance"*

Benjamin Allen's book, *Out of the Ashes, Healing in the AfterLoss*, is a must read for anyone struggling to find hope amidst the kaleidoscope of overwhelming grief. Despite three profound losses, Benjamin shares his journey with remarkable tenderness and offers hope that deep sorrow is not only survivable, but finding a meaningful existence and even joy is quite possible in the afterloss. This book is a compelling addition to grief resources everywhere.
~ Lynda Cheldelin Fell, *International Bestselling Author,*
Producer of Good Grief Talk Show

Grief is not a mental disorder or a disease but a transformative process. Benjamin Allen has written a book that gives people who grieve tools to do the work they need to become what I call fully alive with grief. He does this by sharing his own experience with a wisdom and truth that is born out of his own grief, not out of observing the grief of other people. There is peace as well as pain, joy as well as tears. This is an unwanted journey — one we are sometimes tempted to take alone — but it is better to reach out to the hands that are extended to you. This book is one of those hands.
~ Jan Warner, *Founder of Grief Speaks Out*

OUT of the ASHES

Healing in the AfterLoss

Published by Senssoma Publishing

www.theAfterLoss.com

ISBN 978-0-9915397-1-0

OUT of the ASHES

Healing in the AfterLoss

BENJAMIN SCOTT ALLEN

Dedication

This book is dedicated to everyone that has touched this story and brought it to life and everyone who has been touched by this story and found within these pages a part of themselves.

Contents

Acknowledgments

Nothing lives in isolation. This book is no different for it is the culmination of healing in the shadow of great loss found in the living of life.

First and foremost, Lydia, Matt and Bryan are the ones that have touched these pages the most. It is their story of depth and dignity. This story is a testament to the strength, courage and compassion they lived in the midst of tremendous adversity.

This account of life and loss would not have been possible without Rachel Flower, my wife. She is the one who encouraged me to write my story. She put her heart and soul into every page by editing and re-editing my journey, our journey. She is also the one who relentlessly kept moving this book further along, and ultimately into your hands.

More importantly, Rachel is the one who would sit beside me in my darkest moments. She continues to give me the unconditional support to lean into my sorrow and wander my world of the Afterloss whenever and wherever it leads. It takes a soul of great depth to hold such a space for another and no one has been able to do it better than Rachel.

I would not be alive if it wasn't for my brother, Skip. How do I acknowledge the one who has matched me step for step, shadow for shadow, light for light for my entire life? This book is only a small part of the whole in which I have lived. Yet, for my whole life Skip's love, compassion and wisdom has never wavered. He is a unique man with a unique gift.

I want to thank my father, Jimmy, for supporting the writing of this book from its inception. We all walk through loss differently. He has given me the support to walk where I have needed to go and helped me keep my heart open to the needs of others on this path.

I also want to thank Deborah Brown for her outstanding editing skills, and so much more. As we went through these pages together it was impossible to divorce myself from the reliving of all that I have gone through. Deborah gently helped shape this book as much from her heart as from her skillful professionalism, which is not an easy task, but one for which I am eternally grateful.

Finally, I want to acknowledge you. You probably would not have been drawn to these pages unless there was some loss you have experienced. I want to honor what it takes to lean into sorrow and loss to embrace the preciousness of life. I am grateful that you have chosen to meet me here and I hope you will be able to find comfort in our common path.

OUT of the ASHES

Healing in the AfterLoss

Introduction

This is an account of the common journey within us all. It is a reflection of the universal quest for life's meaning, purpose and for life itself. While my story involves living for many years with a wife and two children with terminal illnesses, we all travel through various life challenges that take us deeper within ourselves. This is where we will meet in our journey. It is a calling from deep to deep, from our common depths into the Afterloss. The world of the Afterloss is a world where what was before is no longer there. Something precious has been lost. It is an after world that needs to find its own time and rhythm. Everyone who has experienced loss knows that world, the one that doesn't fit the world of Before.

We each have our own personal labyrinth in the world of the Afterloss, filled with highs and lows, meaning and meaninglessness, life and death, dishes in the sink and unmade beds. Whether we harbor our days in a cubicle or in the coveted corner office, on the street or in a home, or anywhere in between, we deal with the same inner thoughts, same questions. Who am I? Why am I here? Why is this happening? What is my purpose? We have within each of us the dark places and the yearning for light. It is part of the human condition to yearn for love, to dream, to live in spite of broken dreams, to manage within the slipping of time and the confinement of space.

We hope. We laugh. We cope. We cry. We enter places where we think we are totally alone, where no one can possibly understand, only to discover the paths we walk have so many previous footprints. We are not as alone as we may think. Someone has traveled this path before. What did they find? What am I finding as we share the brevity of our heartbeat and the timelessness of our questions?

Your experience and mine are different, but the same. It is in our sameness that I hope we will meet. Some of you will be able to relate to the external circumstances. There is certainly nothing unique about my journey. Others of you will have your own pathways that have brought you to the places we will explore within these pages.

Come join me in the quest. Perhaps this journey together will unfurl even further the larger context of your life that lies within you. Let us sit together and tell our stories to each other. Find that piece of you that says, "Yes. I know this place. I know what it is like to sit by candlelight and search the flame."

Tell me your story. In the midst of my journey through life and loss, a friend told me a story. It was about a man who had lost his family, his job and his home. The only thing he had left was a rope tied to his neck and he was about to tie the other end to a tree. Another man walked up to him and asked why he was going to end his life. The man said, "I have nothing left." The other man said, "No, that is not true. You have your story."

Can life simply be about shared story? Does the story even matter or is it the collective meaning that binds us? Is our first breath a question mark and if we choose to live life to the fullest can our last breath be an exclamation point?

This is an account of life, not death. Meet me here. Meet me by candlelight and tell me what you have traveled through that brought you to this book. We have not met by accident. I will hear your journey. We will meet deep within this crossroad of your labyrinth and mine, for it is our common story that I speak, and you have already echoed within me. We will share a brief moment before we venture onto our own individual pathways. We will walk away the better because we have shared this moment. No, we are truly not alone.

Welcome. I have been waiting for you.

Part 1:
Living in Loss

Prologue

The swollen sea tossed the dilapidated fishing boat like a cork in a hurricane. The captain, lathered in grease and the smell of old fish, gripped the wheel as the wooden vessel sputtered forward to the crest of the swell and descended into a wall of water. The rain swirled in all directions. I sat in the cabin waiting, too sick to be sick. The captain shouted, "Do what you need to do here. This is as far as we go."

Thirteen years of laughter, slumber parties, movies, bedtime stories, hugs and kisses rested in a thick plastic bag. I reached in with my right hand and pulled out a handful of my child. The ash was devoured by the salt-water swell. With my left hand, I repeated the ritual with the ash of my eight-month-old, a life denied laughter, slumber parties, movies... but full of hugs and kisses.

The captain poured all the weight of his boat's engines toward land. I sat in the cabin, drenched with salt water, cold rain and warm tears. A film of wet ash covered each hand and I stared into the lives of my children. The storm still cried its indignation as I stepped off the boat and walked to the end of the pier. I dipped my hands into the cold, cold sea and watched the ashes drift slowly away. It was my last act as a father.

"Hello, This is Papa ..."

What is the first act of a father? When does a relationship with a child really begin? When does it end? The relationship with my unknown child solidified long before his body entered the world. Many times I would rub Lydia's stomach and in a soft, singing cadence say to our child, "Hello, this is Papa, and I love you."

Just weeks before, Lydia and I sat on the steps of the small, red brick parsonage. We had worked hard that day decorating our child's bedroom, masking the white concrete walls with brightly colored hot air balloons. It was our first real home, even though it still belonged to the church I had just started to pastor. She sat on the first step and I rested on the last of the three, close to her stomach, close to our child. The moon was full that night. It hung over the hill that separated Pacifica from the rest of the San Francisco Bay Area. We shared the dream of our coming days, laughed and joked at our good fortune to find this church, this home, this child.

It was not unlike the first time Lydia and I sat together on the front lawn of her apartment in Fort Worth, Texas, in 1978; the first night we knew we'd be spending other nights together. She was in theological training at Southwestern Baptist Theological Seminary. She was already a nurse, but she had decided to go overseas as a medical missionary. I was in my junior year at Baylor University. I was in Fort Worth to attend a student convention; and since she was like a big sister to me, she offered me a place to spend the night.

Lydia and I first met when I was eleven. She, being three years older, only gave me the courtesy of friendship. Not that I was in love with her then. I fell in love with Lydia the night we shared our laughter on her front lawn. We laughed and laughed that night. Not just giggles, but real belly laughs that leave warm embers on a memory. We were married a year later and set our sights on California, seminary and then only God knew.

And only God did know under the California night of that full moon. I stroked her stomach and sang in a familiar cadence, "Hello, this is Papa, and I love you." Every morning I sang, "Hello, this is Papa, and I love you." Coming home after work I would repeat our ritual. This night was no different from other nights, or at least that is what we thought. Only God knew, but we laughed and talked as if we knew too.

It was a Sunday, three weeks before the due date. I taught a Sunday school class in the small church and preached the morning sermon. Lydia taught a Sunday school class. Lydia and I went home that Sunday afternoon. She wasn't feeling well. She had scaled back her work at St. Mary's Hospital to half time, but she was getting more tired as the birth approached. She stayed home that night when I returned to the church to teach a training class and preach the Sunday night sermon.

It was about ten when her headache started. At eleven thirty she began to vomit. By midnight we were heading for Mt. Zion Hospital in San Francisco, the hospital we had carefully selected in our search for the best place to have our child.

Her attending physician didn't come to the hospital to meet us. Instead, a resident checked her over. Around two in the morning we were sent home, medication in hand.

Exhausted, I locked my eyes on the broken white lines. We entered a tunnel on the highway home. Intermittent lights flashed in sporadic rhythms to illuminate the cab. Still my eyes measured the edge of the hood to the white line leading home.

I felt Lydia's hand slap me across the face. I jerked my head in her direction. Her eyes were rolled back. Blood dripped from her mouth. Her hands curled as they flailed against the window and the dashboard. I pressed her back against the seat with one hand, holding the wheel with the other. The lights of the tunnel quickly flashed – light, dark, light, dark. I screamed her name. No response. The exit on the other side of the tunnel did not smoothly U-turn back to the hospital we had left twenty minutes earlier. But laid out before us was Mary's Help Hospital in Daly City. I held her with one hand and sped the car to the front door of the emergency room, nearly crashing into glass. Attendants burst out the sliding doors. She was still convulsing when they strapped her on the gurney and whisked her away.

I could see her in the other room as they tried to control her flailing arms. She catapulted off the bed and landed hard against the mattress. They wouldn't let me in the room and ultimately closed the door.

The waiting room was empty. I paced the cold white florescent hallway alone. I gripped my chest, slid down the hallway wall and prayed, "God, don't let her die. Please, don't let her die."

In that moment, I felt it wasn't just up to God. Lydia, deep within the multi-layers of life, beyond the surface of consciousness, had a choice to make. She was standing on a precipice undetectable to the human eye. My prayer turned to her, "Please, Lydia, please don't die."

Does God answer prayer? Was I even a player that night or in the days that lay ahead? I sat on the cold tiles in that empty hallway, waiting.

Lydia and I stood a room apart, her life shredded in layers, our child's life in the balance. I stood at the edge of where I'd been, but could not go that night. This was her journey.

My prayers may have echoed into the inner chambers, but even to this day I do not know why what happened happened, nor can I begin to comprehend the interplay of destiny and desire. To this day I wonder what part Lydia played just one room away.

Her physician entered the waiting room. He said he wanted to take her back to Mt. Zion. The seizures had stopped. They said they wanted to induce labor rather than perform a caesarean. Hours of waiting ensued. Her dilation was slow, but she remained in a stable condition.

On October 4, 1982, just this side of midnight, our son, Matthew Benjamin Allen, slid down the birth canal, the umbilical cord wrapped around his neck three times. The attendants unwrapped the cord and rushed Matt to the corner of the room to check his vitals. He was alive. Weak, but alive. They said they would have to take him down to the intensive care for a routine check.

I held Lydia's hand. Was I to go with Matt? Was I to stay with Lydia? I had not slept in over twenty-four hours, but I was clearly awake to the measure of that moment. I looked at Lydia. She was stable. I squeezed her hand, kissed her cheek and followed the tiny gurney that carried our child to the infant intensive care. Once Matt had stabilized I returned to Lydia's room and waited.

They brought our baby to the room. Wrapped snugly in a blanket he descended to his mother's side. His mouth pressed against her nipple in the dance of mother and child. It took only a minute or two before Matt took his first swallows of his mother's milk. It could have been that moment, or maybe another moment when in the womb, which took his life thirteen years later.

Matt went back to the regular nursery after the feeding and I stayed with Lydia. Later, the pediatrician entered Lydia's room and said Matt had to be taken back to the intensive care. He said Matt might not make it through the night, and added: "We are not sure what he has, but I need to tell you he is probably one of the sickest babies in there."

I sat next to our son under the lights of the intensive care. Lydia was too weak to join us. He was covered with sticky plastic circles that held the various monitors on his chest. The ventilator pushed air into his lungs, but still he heaved for every breath. I matched the rhythm of his short breaths and prayed. His left hand gripped my index finger. I leaned close to his ear and softly sang, "Hello, this is Papa, and I love you."

Matt squeezed my finger. This was the final key that unlocked all of me, leaving me utterly defenseless. It was the first of many lessons Matt gave me in the brevity of thirteen years.

Up until then, there was never a time when I let myself completely love. There was always a part of me that held back, safe from complete annihilation, just in case the love I gave was to be lost. With the squeeze of my son's hand I was undone, frighteningly free to love another unconditionally. The only way I can describe it, rather awkwardly, is "I was unable not to love."

Matt fought to live through the night. His bowel wall had broken, probably due to feeding too early after the traumatic birth. He would need an operation to remove three quarters of his bowel and he would have a stoma, a hole in his side, where he would excrete his stool.

Seven days after Matt entered the world, a knife entered him. Lydia was back in the hospital. She came home for a day, continued to bleed and had to return to the hospital for a D&C. I sat by her hospital bed and we waited to know if our son was going to live. The doctor entered with the news. The operation was a success. Hopefully, the remaining bowel would heal enough that in seven months the doctor could reconnect the two sides and he would no longer need the stoma.

The doctor left the room. I hugged Lydia and jubilantly said, "We get to keep him." That was my mantra for the rest of the day. Over and over I thanked God and muttered to myself, "We get to keep him." What I didn't know was how long that would be.

A Knowing in the Unknown

Tomorrow was a long time ago. Linear motion began to erode. The definition of "moment" now was a day, a year, a lifetime, and a breath – anything that leaves a shadow or a mark on time. We did not know it, but we had already started our journey into the Afterloss, that world where all that was before was never to be again. Loss was disguised and lingering in the shadow of our hope. We did not know that the day of his birth was the watershed moment that marked the day three people would die.

Matthew filled our moments. One of us tried to be with him at all times during his first month of life in the intensive care. We were taught how to care for the stoma, how to work with his intolerance to protein and his "failure to thrive." Matt was always hungry. Due to the lack of bowel he needed food practically every hour, on the hour. The food traveled so fast that thirty minutes after eating he produced stool. The acid from the stool broke down the skin around his side. He cried from the pain; the crying made him hungry again.

Day and night the cycle of food, pain, waking, brief intervals of sleep ruled our home. We hung on, hoping the next operation would change the sleepless shifts we shared.

Lydia returned home after her second trip to the hospital and was not much better. She was constantly weary. We put it down to sleepless nights and the intensity of Matt's needs. But Lydia knew. She was deeply in touch with her body and could feel something within her was different and ominous. Her weariness was too weary, her lack of strength too obvious. She told me how, when taking Matt for his regular checkups, she would have to leave an hour early, just so she could find a parking place close enough to the doctor on the crowded streets of San Francisco. Lydia began to measure time by the energy it took.

She leaned against the kitchen counter one day, her arms folded, knees locked for support. She wore her thick brown hair shoulder length in those days. Her small frame had already returned to her pre-pregnant days. Deep brown eyes, usually rich in expression, were dull with weariness. She said, "I feel like something has died inside of me. Something has happened."

Something had happened. A knowing always shadowed our uncertainty.

I never forgot that moment when she spoke those words. Nor did I forget the moment in her long labor when the obstetrician asked me to come into the hallway. She said to me, "We want to give Lydia some platelets. It is just a precaution. She has lost a lot of blood and if we need to do an emergency caesarean she will need them."

I didn't even know what platelets were. The doctor explained the blood clotting effect of platelets. "She could bleed to death without them." I nodded and said, "Do whatever you need to do."

I don't know why I would specifically remember that conversation over the other medical jargon I heard in the hours before Matt's birth. But I do.

Before Lydia and I left for California, in the first year of our marriage, Lydia had a dream. This, too, I remember. It was a dream that shook her to her core. She said, "I was in a large room, like a theater. It was crowded with people. The show ended and we were led to one particular exit. We moved, close together, down this long corridor. I don't know how I know, but I realized we were moving to our deaths. Like we were being led to a gas chamber or something."

I never forgot her dream. Nor did she.

Lydia was strong, powerful in herself and her beliefs. Her wisdom was like her life, not flashy, not pretentious. When she spoke, she had something to say. But she didn't need to speak for those in her presence to experience her depth of spirit. When the "something had died" in her began to take her life, from the first moment to the last, Lydia stood grounded in a serene strength. Even when she cried, her tears ran from deep, still waters. She was, above all, a realist, but during that period we were missing the one piece of reality that carved the rest of our lives.

We didn't know that on October 4, 1982 Lydia had received a transfusion of platelets that carried HIV. We didn't know that the reason Matt's "failure to thrive" was not because he was unable to absorb nutrients. The true reason was that he too was infected by HIV, possibly from the milk that broke through his bowel wall and entered his bloodstream. And we didn't know that destiny was to take the life of one more before it was through.

But we knew something had died; we just didn't know what. Astronomers look into the far reaches of space and detect an imploded star by the orbits of the planets in its gravitational pull. From October 4, 1982 we lived in the gravitational pull of an unknown disease.

We did not miss the signs; we misread the signs. We listened to the multitude of experts. One "expert" literally laughed at Lydia when she told him how many vitamin supplements she was giving Matt. He said, "Matt's urine could care for half of Africa with that amount of vitamins."

But Lydia knew. She had thrown herself headlong into the care of her child. She knew something was wrong. When she asked Matt's pediatrician if Matt could have been infected with this new virus going around San Francisco in 1982, he said, "It is highly unlikely. Practically impossible."

But she knew, not that it was HIV, but "something had died" inside her and something was killing our son.

There are two things I would never do – stand in between a grizzly bear and her cub, and get in the way of Lydia when she was on a mission. The care of Matt was Lydia's mission. She studied medical journals, checked into alternative health and toured the "experts" looking for answers to Matt's physical fragility. Apparently, doctors have to earn the respect of nurses, and this was certainly the case with Lydia. She didn't roll over and give way to the experts. We may not have known what Matt had, but Lydia knew the limitations of doctors. And when it came to the medical world, not one of my favorite terrains to begin with, I stayed out of Lydia's laser-like path.

My path was to sit under the tutelage of this infant that was my son. The nights in the intensive care brought my early lessons. He was strapped to machines and monitors, but the wires stretched to the rocking chair and to the beating of my heart. I would rock him, sing softly in the crowded room, and talk to him of the days I thought lay ahead of us. "We got to keep him." The night he lived through, the operation that was a success, the steadying of his breath and his slow recovery was my gift. And that gift was never lost on me. Never.

The day we were able to bring him home I carried him to his room, the tiny bedroom full of hot air balloons. A balloon mobile drifted over his second-hand crib as I lowered him down on his bed for the first time. His dark brown eyes briefly scanned the room before closing.

That night, Lydia insisted we read him a book. "Read him a book?" I said. "He's only a month old!"

She picked a book with thick pages. "It doesn't matter. We are going to read to him every night."

We read the book, sharing every other page.

Born of Spirit into the Unknowable

The movement of spirit takes its own course. Spirit has always been a part of my life. I was taught from an early age that spirit was as real as my body. It was simply part of the landscape. No matter what the scenery, it was through the lens of spirit that I was taught to see life's unfolding mysteries.

My earliest lesson in spirit clothed an ominous foreboding that spoke of the years to come. I wonder sometimes whether the mysteries that stream through the present tense are simply an understanding of the past.

I was four. My two older brothers had already moved into the academic realm of first and third grade. I spent most of my days alone without other children. In the backyard next to the garage wall was a long pile of wood, four stacks high. That woodpile was my battleship, my stagecoach, my rocket ship, anything and everything my little imagination could fantasize. For hours on end I would travel the high seas in search of pirates, soar into space to do battle with aliens, and ride my stagecoach through desert plains fighting bad guys. My sidekick, first mate and all around best friend was Little Bit, our Boston Terrier dog. We were inseparable. The Lone Ranger had Tonto. I had Little Bit.

One day I heard a fire engine siren out in front of our little suburban street. I rushed to the high wooden gate, undid the latch and hurried to the front yard to watch this big red truck soar pass. I was captivated by the sounds, the size of the machine, the speed. After the fire truck dipped down the hill and out of sight, I turned to Little Bit to speak of our latest adventure. No doubt the woodpile was about to be transformed into the biggest, brightest fire engine in the world.

Little Bit was gone. It had to be the noise that scared him. He had never left my side before.

For three days my family and I looked for my dog. I had left the gate open. It was my fault. I felt the weight of what I had done.

On the third day, my older brother, Skip, age six, came running up to me. Skip was the protector of the family. The middle of three boys, he was the one that ran interference, watched out for me and carried the weight of light and shadow that all families seem to collect along the way. Skip, in his usual dramatic fashion, said, "Whatever you do don't look in the box in the garage."

Compliance has never been one of my stronger qualities. I heeded his warning long enough to see him run off to his next urgent responsibility.

The brown cardboard box was in the corner of the garage, pushed against a few rakes and the lawnmower. I truly did not know what I was to find. Innocence has its advantages.

It was Little Bit's open eyes I saw first. To a four-year-old, open eyes means awake; but these eyes were empty. Even before I scanned her crushed body, I knew. For the first time I saw eyes devoid of spirit. All I could see was that my dog was dead. And the eyes, those empty eyes, weren't the eyes of my constant companion that licked my face every morning, ate half my sandwiches and fought the forces of evil from our woodpile in the backyard. Those weren't her eyes.

I buried my tears in my pillow for three days, not leaving my room. I had killed my dog. Skip kept a vigil over me. Even though it was his dog too, he stood watch over me. It was my next lesson in spirit. No spirit travels this dream alone. Interwoven in the layers of moment is spirit's collectiveness. My father, the Southern Baptist minister, performed the service. The neighbors next door laughed as the family stood around the broken ground in the backyard. Prayers were said to Jesus. Scriptures read. The Gates of Heaven invoked to comfort. But heaven was someplace else. Somewhere Little Bit was, and I wasn't.

We covered Little Bit with fresh dirt. It was my first funeral. The experience that has lingered long into this dream I live today is that, for me, funerals don't help.

Empty and Full

Our second son, Bryan Caleb Allen, was born on May 13, 1985. We had moved to Colorado the year before. Lydia was working part-time as a psychiatric nurse and I was the youth minister at First Christian Church, Colorado Springs.

Bryan was a fighter. He had to be. He was three months premature. Lydia had major complications and needed a caesarean. I held her hand, but I chose not to look over the sheet into her torn womb.

Bryan spent the first three weeks of his life in the intensive care unit. There were complications, unknown complications. His heart pulsated in irregular rhythms. It was touch and go. Lydia was again physically decimated.

Bryan's eyes were deep blue and reflected an aged wisdom. He was beautifully proportioned from head to toe. That's what I counted first — his toes. I just wanted normalcy.

When they said he was going to have to go to the intensive care unit my heart crumbled. Someone once said, "It is not the future we fear the most. Our greatest fear is that the past will repeat itself."

It was the smell of the antiseptic soap that took me back two years earlier. It was the coarseness of the brush that we used to scrub our fingers before we could touch our child that catapulted me back there again. It was the paper mask that collected the sweat and recycled my breaths that left me only one step away from what I so desperately never wanted to experience again.

Again, I held the small hand of another son. I watched him heave for every breath. Again, there were the smells of the intensive care unit, of children struggling to live. Watching parents waiting on the precipice of life and death praying for miracles filled me, emptied me, and ripped me to shreds.

Bryan's eyes were empty and full at the same time. There was something already lost in him. We believed that if we could get him through the first days, he would make it, just like Matt made it. Again, Lydia and I took turns in our familiar vigil.

Lydia bonded with Bryan in the way I had bonded with Matt. Maybe it was the unconscious common path that drew them into that layer of life, a layer deep and still. I saw immediately the uniqueness of their interwoven spirits. Bryan had the same tenacity as Lydia, the inner strength to do what was necessary. He was calm and determined. His breathing was not desperate and driven like Matt's first days. Bryan's breathing was steady and rhythmic, strong and defiant. I knew from the first, this child was Lydia's child. And I believed he would live because he was Lydia's child.

It was ironic. Bryan physically looked like me. Matt physically looked like Lydia. But the reflection of Matt's spirit was more of me, and Bryan's spirit was to Lydia like the reflection of the moon on a still pond.

We all collected wisdom from Bryan's short life, but it was Lydia that reached the furthest into the presence of Bryan. Lydia's inner knowing met Bryan's inner being in a place where spirit moves deepest in the mysteries.

Bryan came home with a heart monitor. Lydia laid Bryan in his bed I placed the monitor in the corner of the crib. Bryan's room was dressed in bright, colorful rainbows. His eyes surveyed the room; whenever he saw his big brother, Bryan stopped and locked his strong gaze on Matt.

We were told his heart would grow stronger. It did, and the monitor was abandoned after three or four weeks. But Bryan did not grow stronger. He, too, had this strange phenomenon of "failure to thrive." He, like Matt, made the rounds of medical experts.

Lydia's recovery was slow. No one on the outside really knew the degree of her deterioration. She never complained and when anyone entered our world she would rise to the occasion. If asked, she downplayed her condition. Her focus was on Bryan.

Matt still wasn't sleeping through the night. This was at two and half years. Bryan slept more out of exhaustion, and so did Lydia and I.

We braced ourselves every morning for the day ahead. But we were unable to brace ourselves for the call.

I picked up the phone. The woman on the other end asked for Lydia. She said she was with the blood bank in San Francisco. I handed Lydia the phone. She sat down on the couch. I stood next to her and watched. Lydia asked questions. "What do you mean? What kind of tests? What's it for?"

I don't remember the length of the conversation. I do remember the length of the moment when Lydia said, "The donor that gave me the blood at Matt's birth has died of AIDS. They want us all to be tested."

Defining Moments

Bryan had just turned four months. Matt was less than three weeks from his third birthday. Lydia was twenty-eight years old, I was twenty-five.

Time – the luxury of illusion. And before the phone call broke the illusion, there was time.

In the days that unfolded from the phone call nothing felt real. We put the pieces together as best we could. All the doctors, hospitals and mysteries slotted into place. The unknown condition became knowable, but we still knew so little.

Lydia's obstetrician tested us and the boys were going to be tested by their pediatrician. Lydia was already there with the boys by the time I arrived at the pediatrician's office. We waited in the outer office, clothed in secrecy and fear.

Our radar was now keenly attuned to any broadcast or story about AIDS (it wasn't till years later when the term HIV became the standard name, but for consistency I would rather just use the term HIV). Rock Hudson kissed Linda Evans on Dynasty and the big question was whether Linda was going to get HIV, too. A child in Indiana, Ryan White, was forced out of school and ostracized. A five-year-old with HIV in Atascadero, California bit another child on the playground and mayhem ensued. A family's house in Florida was burned to the ground because three of their children were infected.

We sat in the waiting room with the other parents and their children; Matt and I played with the multi-colored toys in the corner. Lydia held Bryan as he slept. And we pretended everything was normal; pretended *we* were normal.

When we left the doctor's office to wait for the test results, we knew. Lydia and I set the children in the two cars. She strapped Bryan in his car seat in her car. I sat Matt in my car. We pulled out of the parking lot, one following the other.

I drove the four-lane road by remote control. Matt looked out the window. At the stoplight I looked at Lydia in the lane next to me. She looked at Bryan as he sat between us. Then her eyes rose to meet mine.

There are moments, defining moments. There are words, inadequate words. And there are distances, indefinable distances.

I wanted to hold her, to jump out of the car and wrap her in my arms. We pleaded into each other's eyes. She looked into the backseat at Matt. She looked back at me. The light changed. And we went back to pretending.

All the tests were done; the results came back. Lydia, Matt and Bryan were HIV positive. My test came back negative. The distance I felt at the stoplight grew even further. It was best described in an article by a woman dying of cancer. She beautifully articulated her experience of how when someone is moving towards death with a terminal illness there are some places others who have not experienced this simply cannot go. I could walk alongside Lydia, but not within her path. On one level we worked in harmony to bring as much normalcy to Matt's and Bryan's lives as possible, but in one of the layers buried beyond the surface, the severing of paths was inevitable.

Lydia's nature was to move with steady, uncompromising determination due to her innate capacity to love. My father, who knew her well, once said of Lydia during her teenage years, "Lydia would be the president of the Wounded Bird Society if there was one." She took her spiritual beliefs seriously. She was brought up in a conservative Southern Baptist home, Christian to the core. She was not fanatical in her theology, but the roots of her faith ran deep. She lived her beliefs in social justice and the protection of the disenfranchised.

Now we had joined the disenfranchised. More importantly, our children were in danger of being the target of the hysteria that gripped the country in 1985. Cries for the quarantine of "those people" reached a crescendo in the right-wing Christian America. The HIV-infected were moral degenerates, rightfully condemned to death for their sins according to the keepers of the faith. Under the banner of righteous holiness came a tidal wave of hate and fear.

It was Lydia's strength, determination and quiet depth that stabilized the chaos within and around us. I was ready to fight the world – win, lose or draw. It was Lydia who taught me the power of softness. She steadied us in those initial days. When she cried in my arms, she cried from the expanse, not shrinking self-pity, but from that part of the stream that widens into an ocean.

When the obstetrician circulated Lydia's records with her name on it to all the hospital staff that attended Bryan's birth, Lydia was angry, but she moved with a methodical calm. That was her way. When I met with the senior minister of the church and told him that Lydia, Matt and Bryan were HIV-infected and I was negative, he asked for my resignation. Lydia shook her head and said, "Let's take the boys to the park."

We sat on the swings in the cool Colorado autumn. Matt was bundled in a ski jacket, playing on the jungle gym. Bryan was wrapped in blankets in the portable basinet. Softly Lydia and I drifted on the swings, suspended above the dirt. She laid her head against the chain, gently twisting from left to right. Her voice was soft, subdued. "What are we going to do now?"

The church set up a meeting with the parents of Matt's Sunday school class. We feared the worst. I had already been offered a mandatory severance package. We worked through our diminishing options.

The parents' meeting ended. We waited for the response. There wasn't one. We thought surely someone would call to tell us what happened. Our minds went in all directions except the most probable one.

The people of the church were basically shocked. Good people not knowing what to do. One person told me years later that they didn't know what the staff and board had done. They thought there would be time to offer love and support.

But in the silence we felt shut off and shunned. And we, too, shut off and shunned. Out of fear we fled, packed all our belongings and left Colorado. Good people not knowing what to do.

Making a Home Out of a House

In a rented truck holding everything we had, I drove for 15 hours from Colorado Springs to Fort Worth, Texas, to be close to family. Lydia and the boys were already there. The meter was running on the truck rental and Lydia had yet to find a home. Where were we to find a home when homes of people with HIV were being burned to the ground? Who would rent to us? Who was Matt going to play with if and when the parents in the neighborhood found out? Would we be so lucky to get the silent treatment again? Texas wasn't exactly a hotbed of liberal generosity.

We found a house. A friend of my father had a rental property and she took the chance and rented it to us.

Two children lived next door. What would happen if they knew? How were we going to explain why Bryan was on an oxygen tube? Why Bryan was almost six months old and still only five and half pounds?

The biggest dancing act was to explain why we never let Matt play next door. Why the kids always had to come to our house. Lydia and I had decided from the beginning that one of us, or someone that knew about Matt's condition, would always be with him. Universal precautions, the proper handling of blood, were not the norm in 1985.

Matt was too young to understand what he should do if he fell and bled so we were on constant alert, watching, just in case.

This need always to be present with Matt made his socialization difficult. I lived in utter terror thinking something was going to happen to him. Lydia knew no fear. She enrolled Matt in a playgroup for three-year-olds where the mothers were present. When I was off at work she packed up Bryan, oxygen tank and all, dressed Matt, and took him every week to be with other children.

We tried to find churches that would accept Matt. We told the senior ministers of Matt's condition and asked if he could attend Sunday school. Most turned us down. One church actually voted in a staff meeting to ask us not to come. One minister said I could take Matt to the class and stay with him. The Sunday school teacher didn't know Matt or why I hung around. It was more than uncomfortable for both of us as I lingered in the room pretending it was normal. That only lasted two weeks and we gave up.

I would take Matt to fast food chains where there was a playground just so he could be with other kids. One time Matt came running up to me with great excitement and said, "I made a new friend!"

"You did?" I said, matching his wide eyes. "What's his name?"

"I don't know! I'll go ask him!"

I was able to smile just long enough for Matt to turn and run back into the crowd of children. Matt didn't know the difference between a friend and an acquaintance. I had already learned how to let my tears flow on the inside and not down my cheeks. I sat watching Matt play with another stranger, crying, wondering if he would ever have friends.

We searched everywhere for friends for Matt. We shared our plight with Dr. Janet Squires, Matt's pediatrician in Fort Worth. She listened to us unload our dilemma. Then she said, "You can bring Matt over to our house. I have three small children and he can play with them."

Janet legitimized the socialization of our son. Her young children playing alongside our son gave us strength, a place to stand in the midst of a world where we felt isolated and in fear of reprisal.

If Matt could play with her children, maybe other children would befriend him.

It was Lydia's natural propensity to "hold her cards close to her chest," but she rose to a level beyond belief. I was never that astute. Before *the call*, I would tell the world everything, pour out my soul. Lydia taught me the "art of discretion." She was cool under fire. Anyone would look at Lydia and never know the sorrow she bore, the physical and emotional pain she endured, the crushing weight of loss she carried.

I recently read about a fireman out in a burnt forest who found three baby birds still alive. Their mother had covered the three babies with her body. She could have flown away, but she chose to stay, to die for her young. That was Lydia. Every day she felt the fire that engulfed us and she stayed forever vigilantly perched over her young.

One day Lydia and I were talking at the kitchen counter. Matt was facing the other way eating a sandwich at the table. We were calmly talking in code about our present trials and tribulations. I quietly said to Lydia, "I'm just sick of all the hassles."

Without turning around Matt lightheartedly said, "What hassles?"

Lydia and I looked at each other and laughed. From then on, when the density of a moment became crushing, Lydia and I would look at each other and say, "What hassles?"

Changing Bandages

Bryan never crawled, never held his head up on his own, and never grew past the size of an infant in his brief eight and half months. He spent his days in pain. A central line pierced his chest and the plastic tube lodged in an artery to his heart. We took turns cleaning and changing the bandage that kept the tube clean.

Lydia taught me how to pull the clear plastic bandage off the white gauze. She guided me in how to clean off the old antiseptic. The brown liquid swab on a long plastic stick was carefully drawn out of the disposable paper package. Even the rubber gloves were not to touch what was to touch his skin. Carefully I would encircle the tube only once with that portion of the brown swab, turn the stick and make another circle just wider than the last. Then I would place new white sterile gauze over the tube to Bryan's heart, ending with the clear plastic tape that held the central line steady.

Bryan was usually expressionless while I went through the routine. His large blue eyes followed my voice as we chatted during the process. Actually, I chatted. He spent most of his energy just working on one breath to the next. His life force was weak, but his eyes stayed focused and strong. He had the most intense, knowing eyes I've ever seen.

One day Lydia was off with Matt. It was my turn to change the bandage on Bryan's central line. I was chattering along letting my voice wash over him. His eyes were locked on me. The clamp that held the central line came off. Blood began to pour out on the changing table. I looked for the clip. I tried to hold the tiny tube closed with my rubber-gloved hand to no avail. Blood, precious blood, from his little body continued to flow out on the table. I put my finger over the end of the tube. My heart stopped. My glove had touched so many unsterile items in the procedure. Anything could have been on the end of that glove. I found the clamp, sealed the tube and finished the job.

I held Bryan in the rocking chair wondering if my panic was going to kill him. I waited the coming days looking for signs of a new infection. I held Bryan from spirit to spirit with skin to skin, but the distance between journeys was what held us closest.

The Pulsing of a Heart

Most parents teach their children how to live. We had to teach Matt and Bryan how to die. Lydia and I were forced into seeing death as a natural part of life, even for an eight-month-old and a three-year-old. In September 1985 we were novices. Lydia and I stumbled through the darkness of our days doing the best we could. But in the years from 1985 to Matt's death in 1995 I attempted to make the transition of life to death as just another part of this whole planetary experience. I tried to prepare a three-year-old for the inevitable death of his brother. On a psychological level Lydia and I tried to make going to the hospital to see Bryan as common as going to the park. But we would meet Matt on whatever layer he chose to engage. The balancing of layer upon layer and moving in the rhythm of a three-year-old was a challenge. Nevertheless, we were keenly aware that whatever we reflected in Bryan's life would profoundly affect Matt's capacity to weave the death of his mother, and his own death, into the finer, subtler layers in which we resided.

The last months of Bryan's life were filled with pain. Lydia and Janet, his doctor, felt the best approach to Bryan's care was to give him as much pain medication as he could handle without sending him over the edge. Bryan received the meds every four hours and the pain subsided for about an hour. Lydia and I would take turns holding him in his most painful moments, exhaustion would relieve us all, and some of that time Bryan would sleep. Then the cycle would begin again. I asked Lydia why she didn't want to give Bryan more pain meds. She said, "Because it might hurt his brain development."

I said, "Lydia, he's dying. What brain development?"

That was when I realized the depth of the bond she had with Bryan. She was not yet able to let him go.

On my shift, holding him in his conscious agony, I would rock him in the chair. He would cry and scratch into my chest. I sang to him, like I sang to Matt, and rocked, like I rocked Matt. I visualized love encircling Bryan. I'd slowly stroke his soft head and sing. I would visualize this love being so deep and all encompassing that when Bryan died he would know this love. He would enter the next realm knowing everything he needed in order to live in rhythmic harmony with that dimension. The pulsating heartbeat of life wouldn't miss a beat when Bryan died. I kept seeing Bryan look around at his new surroundings after death and say, "I know this place. I felt this in my father's arms."

૱૦૱

It was the day before Bryan was to die. He was in the hospital again. Lydia and I had this routine that when one of the boys was in the hospital one of us would stay with him at all times. We made every effort to provide stability and continuity.

I had just returned from a business trip the night before. We were in Bryan's hospital room when Janet came in to talk to us about Bryan's present condition. All his tests were on the positive side. He was stable and his tests looked good, better than they had looked for a long time. Lydia hung on Janet's every word.

Lydia was exhausted. She was immune-compromised as it was and I convinced her to come home to sleep. It would be the first time we were able to sleep together in a long time. And the first time Bryan was to sleep alone.

Lydia, Matt and I were dressed early that Sunday morning when the phone call came. Lydia answered the phone and Janet said we needed to get to the hospital right away. I drove the empty roads as fast as I could. Lydia looked out the window in silence. We rushed to Bryan's hospital floor. She went straight into his room while I took Matt down to the playroom. With Matt well situated I rushed to the room and opened the door. Lydia turned from the crib to me. Bryan's limp body lay on her chest; she was stroking his head, just like she had done a thousand times. She looked into my eyes and before I made it through the door and said, "He's dead."

She rested her head on Bryan's and rocked him in the familiar soft rhythm. I wrapped one arm around her, one arm around Bryan and kissed him on the top of his small head. His body was still warm. He had just died.

We took turns holding him. I held him in my lap and felt his body draining of warmth. There, on the edge of eternity, we both lingered. I felt Bryan's presence. It was not the presence of an eight-month-old child. His soul was ancient, soft and gentle. He stayed to sorrow for me, to comfort, to explain. He was free now to answer me. His little body lay in my lap and I felt him stroke my soul as I stroked an empty child. I sensed his understanding. He understood better than I the chasm we endured in this dimension.

For the first time, but not the last, I was guided into the gift of death. I felt a piece of me move with him into layer upon layer, to the source, to where the Unknown knows. And I was gifted with a part of him in the exchange. Maybe it is always there, I don't know. But I do know we embraced in an understanding, a moment, a dream within the dream. I do know that as his body grew cold, he clothed me in softness. And I do know he didn't miss a beat. He knew love. He stepped into the familiar. He waited to tell me of the pulsating heartbeat of Spirit.

Almost six months passed before Lydia and I talked about the moments of Bryan's leaving. She said she had the same experience. Bryan had waited to say goodbye to her, too.

He waited to touch us when we were no longer able to touch him.

The reason it took time to discuss Bryan's day of death was because I carried the weight of asking Lydia to come home that night. Lydia never blamed me. I did. She was not the kind of person who would tear into another to find a way to block her own pain. Lydia faced pain like no other I've met. She truly owned her journey.

I felt regret, not guilt, for convincing Lydia to come home that night. For I believe Bryan needed the space to die. Lydia and Bryan were so intertwined.

Death takes a certain degree of solitude in order to experience the expanse. Bryan, the ancient one, needed that time to tear away from time.

Lydia couldn't let Bryan go. And Bryan wouldn't go until she could.

They kept Bryan's body in the hospital room while we went home to retrieve the clothes in which he was to be buried. The mortician, a friend of the family, agreed to bring the casket to the room. We wanted to place Bryan in the casket ourselves.

We dressed Bryan in a dark blue sailor suit with a white collar. The small casket was a light metallic blue. The mortician, well-versed in moments like this, patiently waited outside. When we were ready he entered the room. I lowered Bryan's body into the casket. The lid was about to close. All three of us noticed that Bryan's head wasn't sitting straight on the pillow. The mortician instinctively reached down to straighten Bryan's head, but before touching him he froze and recoiled. Lydia straightened Bryan's head and we closed the casket. It was the last time we saw our son's body.

Lydia felt the mortician had recoiled because of the HIV. There were so many wild ideas about transmission floating in society at that time and people were scared. We all were saturated with misinformation, increasing our isolation, and our radar was very sensitive to the slightest slight. But I didn't see it that way. This man, who traveled three hours to bring us this casket, who stood in the room with us when many at that time wouldn't, simply wanted to give us the space to prepare our own child. The last look was a psychic photograph, a head tilted for eternity that we could not bear, a memory that had the capacity to haunt or to heal. It was our last chance to do for Bryan, to be parents.

Where's the Cake?

We did not own the grave Bryan was buried in. It belonged to my grandfather. It was an extra one he had lying around, literally. He had three. He had already used his. His wife, riddled with Alzheimer's, waited for hers. And this was a leftover. Before my grandfather died, as his life force was working its way into the beyond, he said to me, "Listen, if that baby dies, I have an extra plot."

We didn't know about the HIV at the time. So, I said, "Thanks, Granddad, but Bryan's going to be fine."

"Well, if he does. It's yours."

Maybe there is a knowing that comes when someone enters that part of the journey. A common language emerges where words become a wasteland. My grandfather knew what I did not.

The grave was in Brownwood, Texas, a three hour drive from Fort Worth. It was a town where I spent my summers with my grandparents, but neither Lydia nor I ever lived there. We had no money and so we accepted the invitation to bury Bryan there.

Lydia, Matt and I drove three hours from our home to where Bryan's body was to lie. Clouds, like sky mountains, cluttered the blue backdrop. The February air was not too cool.

We spoke little as we drove, each listening to our own worlds as we pulled into the flat cemetery.

Friends and family lingered in small groups. No one stood by the casket and there were a few rows of light brown metal chairs. Matt, in his three years and three months, had never seen such an occasion. He skipped along the pathway directly to the front row of metal chairs, right in front of the blue casket he remembered from the hospital. I followed and sat next to him.

In his usual lightheartedness Matt said, "Where's the cake?"

At first I didn't understand. I softly said, "There is no cake, Matt."

The only time Matt had seen a gathering of family and friends like that was at his birthdays. It was his first lesson in funerals. Birthday parties have cake. Funerals don't.

We stayed the night in Brownwood. The next day, Lydia wanted to take Matt back to the grave so our toddler could better conceptualize the finality of never seeing his brother again. I never would have thought of such a thing, just like I never would have thought to start reading a book every night to a one-month-old, but Lydia did. She lived in an inner balance that even the most crushing turmoil couldn't undo. She was in her deepest sorrow, but she said it was important for Matt.

We balanced sorrow and serenity as best we could. The mound over the grave was high; the earth was as unsettled as Lydia and I were. Matt skipped over to the clumps of dirt, loose rocks and gravel. He started taking the pieces of dirt off the mound, throwing them to the side. Again, his light heart didn't hold the weight and he cheerfully said, "Let's take Bryan home now."

Lydia and I looked at each other. She knelt down next to him; her eyes closed as she pressed our son against her chest. She said, "We can't Matt. He's not coming back. He's in heaven."

Matt was just learning to swim. I would take him once a week to the pool for lessons. I bent down next to him as Lydia continued to softly stoke his hair. I said, "Matt, you know how when you swim you take off your shoes?"

Matt nodded.

"That's because when you swim you don't need shoes. You can go faster and it's more fun, right?"

Matt nodded again.

"Well, death is like that. Just like we don't need shoes when we swim, Bryan doesn't need his body where he is now. He can play better and have more fun without it. Just like we can swim and have more fun without shoes. So Bryan left his body here."

It was lame. It certainly didn't touch the enormous metaphysical ramifications of death, yet to a three-year-old, it seemed to work.

But what really worked was the spirit in which Lydia and I moved death into both the ordinary and the inevitable. It was just another part of life. We worked hard to walk the tightrope. We got back in the car for the three-hour drive back to Fort Worth, back to where we had come from, but never to return.

An Honor and a Privilege

Even before we knew about the HIV, Matt and I had already entered something uniquely ours. We loved to laugh. We loved to play. When he was about two he discovered the movie *The Wizard of Oz*. Like all two-year-olds, once is not enough. We watched that movie over and over, and over; each time was like the first time for Matt. The television sat on a cardboard cabinet. We claimed the small space under the TV as our Oz. He always got to be Dorothy and I ended up as Toto for most of our excursions down that yellow brick road. Sometimes I was the Tin Man or the Scarecrow, but Dorothy preferred Toto. I could squeeze my head and a quarter of my chest into Oz. Matt, I mean Dorothy, took up most of the room.

We played games and sang songs. Lydia would teach us new educational songs and we would sing to our hearts' content.

One song was a little rhyme that went through the features of the face. The words were "eyes, ears, nose and mouth..." repeated, it seemed, endlessly. During the song we would touch our eyes, then our ears, the nose and, yes, the mouth.

At the beginning of one of Matt's afternoon naps I lay down next to him, hoping he would sleep. I stayed completely still, pretending to be asleep. Matt softly touched my eye and whispered "eye." I felt his small hand brush against my ear and heard the whisper, "ear." He went through the whole song, his soft voice flowing over me.

Matt studied me and I studied Matt. I was given the gift of being this child's father. I was to teach him, show him the ways of this plane of existence. And Matt, I knew from the very beginning, was to teach me. Even then I knew I was sitting at the small feet of a very large soul.

During the last years of his life I often said to him, "It is an honor and privilege to be your father." He would return, "And it is an honor and privilege to be your son." I wasn't kidding; nor were my words rote or hollow. One night, a month or two before Bryan died, there was a thunderstorm, one of those Texas thunderstorms that explode in the sky and rattle the windows. I didn't want Matt to be scared of thunder. His young life had already been rattled enough. I made every thunderous clap a moment of celebration, every flash of light lifted into excitement. I said, "Matt, let's have a slumber party."

Matt lit up. "Yeah!"

He didn't know exactly what a slumber party was, but he was all for it. So, we folded out the couch. We snuggled under the covers and looked at the show outside our window. We got into a tickling fight, laughing and joking. Lydia walked by and said, "You guys aren't having a slumber party. You're having a rowdy party."

Matt and I looked at each other and burst into laughter. "A rowdy party! Yep, that's what this is!"

It was a Friday night. Friday night from that night to the day he died became rowdy night. Every Friday we would rent a movie, pick up a pizza or something equally unhealthy and pick out a piece of candy that was officially christened our "rowdy snack." We snuggled. We made tents and discovered new worlds.

We made memories.

One of Matt's greatest gifts to me was how he could turn the mundane into mystical magic. And if he were here right now he wouldn't have a clue as to what I'm talking about. He never realized it, but I saw it. I believe every person that encountered Matt walked away better and he never made any effort whatsoever to make it so.

Matt and I were returning from the playground a few blocks from the house one afternoon. I would take him there every day after work. We both looked forward to it and it was a much-needed break for Lydia. We had prepared him for Bryan's inevitable death with a conversation here, an answered question there. But on this occasion we were just doing what we did best—hangin' out.

Matt sat quiet in the car seat next to me. I figured he was just tired from swinging in the swing. On the tire swing I would twirl Matt into the furthest galaxies. We'd pass all the planets, past Pluto, and then sail out into the beyond. Matt wore out easily so it was not unusual for him to silently rest on the way home. He, like his mother, had a natural propensity to use his finite energy wisely.

Out of the blue Matt said, "When I die, Mickey is going to come get me and we're going to dance on the clouds." He was referring to Mickey Mouse, of course.

I acted like I always acted when death was mentioned. I nonchalantly said, "Oh, yeah, that'd be nice. Mickey's a nice guy. I wouldn't mind dancing on the clouds with Mickey myself."

Matt thought for a minute. He looked out the window and said, "Yeah, that'll be nice."

I didn't know how long Matt had to live. It was only three months from the time we got the phone call to Bryan's death. It was the longest three months of my life, but in reality, three months is a millisecond. AZT had yet to arrive as a *maybe* to extend the life of a person with HIV. Lydia was in enormous pain, her energy low. I had to carry her up flights of stairs on several occasions because she was so exhausted. We lived not knowing if Matt's infection or Lydia's physical deterioration would mirror Bryan's. We never knew how long, or rather, how little time we had.

Matt and I returned home. Just like a parent would share with the other parent that their child had added two plus two for the first time I said to Lydia, "Guess what? Matt said that when he died Mickey's going to come get him and they're going to dance on the clouds."

Lydia didn't miss a beat. She bent down and hugged Matt and said, "That's wonderful. I bet Mickey will like that."

It was like the rest of our lives. It was a normal response to an abnormal situation.

The Lens of Spirit

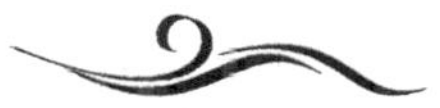

I was taught to look through the lens of Spirit into life from my very first breath. Life and death were natural phenomena, part of life. Even in the womb I was dying, literally. I was an RH-negative baby, which meant my mother's antibodies were attacking me. I was a caesarean birth a few months early, just like Bryan. I spent my first weeks of life in intensive care, just like Matt and Bryan.

There was an experimental procedure in the mid-fifties that entailed a complete blood transfusion. In the first days of life I was washed out and new blood flowed within my frail body. Unfortunately, tests later showed that the blood I received may have transmitted leukemia. For about a year I was taken for a monthly bone marrow test because it was inconclusive as to whether it was leukemia or not. After the first year I still had to take intermittent tests.

I vividly remember one occasion when I was lying on the hospital bed. My mother was there. A medical team in white coats circled the bed. They were about to strap me down in order to stick the needle in my back to draw the blood. One attendant pressed my left arm down and another attendant tried to tie my right arm to the other side. I screamed and kicked, fighting with everything I had.

My mother screamed, too. She screamed at the doctor to let me go. She frantically tried to convince them that if they let me go I would stay still for the procedure. The doctor thought she was crazy. A small child would never stay still as a large needle pierced the bone to draw the marrow. My mother was furious, and fortunately, a very articulate advocate for my cause. I certainly helped by squirming, screaming and making every attempt to bite any arm that might come close enough. The doctor succumbed, reluctantly.

My mother held my hand. I looked into her strong, soft eyes. Then as the needle penetrated my skin and pushed through the bone I closed my eyes, and stayed perfectly still. Without restraint I was able to stay still.

Stillness and movement are the levers of spirit. In all those times I spent alone as a child, I was never alone. There was always the presence of Spirit, and it was the lens in which I viewed life. I spent a lot of time alone to reflect and experience the reflection of spirit.

That's what I always wanted from my earliest remembrances. My home, while not without its challenges, was an easy environment to discover spirit. My father was working for civil rights in the early sixties. In Dallas, Texas, a white Southern Baptist minister working for equality was not the most popular guy in town. My mother's journey was steeped in sorrow and pain – physically, mentally and spiritually. She, like St. John of the Cross, touched that "dark night of the soul." She was in and out of psychiatric wards up until I was eighteen. She spent my junior and senior years of high school in a psychiatric ward in another city. The first year there were no visitors, but the second year I would make the trek to see her.

My mother had a vivacious laugh and a wicked sense of humor. Her heart was as wide and deep as her soul and her eyes were carved by that depth. She was not born to skim on the surface of life.

But while she rose quietly within her pain, my response to pain was to fight. Just as I raged against the doctors that held me down to pierce my bone, I raged against anything that tried to force me into what was not I. Unfortunately, as a teenager, I didn't know me. It was annihilation and reconstruction. I was a walking chemical compound afloat on the sea of alcohol in search of spirit. An overdose at fourteen steered me in one direction. A suicide attempt at sixteen landed me in a mental ward. It was the same ward in which my oldest brother, Michael, had just spent several months after his complete breakdown and diagnosis of schizophrenia. I remembered the psychiatrist saying to me after a few days that I wasn't crazy. I was kind of disappointed when they sent me home after the meds cleared my system. They let me go. No follow-up counseling. No day therapy groups. He said I was a normal kid going through a rough patch. No, I was a normal kid searching for where life truly lives.

There is sometimes a fine line between insanity and mysticism. Michael, four years older than me, crossed that line. At the age of eighteen, Michael's fragmentation opened into a passageway that struggles for congruency between what he sees and where it fits here. I learned a long time ago that I'm no arbiter of what's real and what isn't. But Michael's world is foreign to me, too wide to enter. Michael's world appears to me as a dismembered dream lost in someone else's dream.

Michael and I were never really close. We always seemed to travel parallel universes even as children, only encountering each other in skirmishes and uneasy truces. I never understood Michael. Where my mother's torment was soft, Michael's anguish was jagged and harsh.

Skip's torment was holding in who he was and who he wasn't supposed to be. Skip is gay. The middle son in the middle of a Southern Baptist family in the middle of Dallas, Texas, born in the middle of the 1950s is not an easy trail to blaze. Skip's lens of spirit was skewed by a world that denied him and his authenticity, but his resilient spirit kept him safe and sane.

Near Death, Death Waits

My volatile teenage years reached their ultimate crescendo in a major car accident at the age of twenty. On a two-lane country road outside of San Antonio, Texas, I met the hood of my car, the windshield and my Maker. A drunk swerved his car into my lane, then back into his and at the last moment, back into mine, hitting my car head on.

When he first turned the corner in the distance I said to myself, "I'm going to die." The entire event, except for the very last second, was in slow motion. Peace. Pure peace encircled me as he moved from lane to lane.

In the last second I fell out of timelessness back into time and turned the wheel sharply to the right. I turned the car just enough for the left side of the hood to buckle first and smash against the windshield. My head was coming in the other direction. The hood of the car and my forehead kissed at the glass simultaneously. He was going seventy-five miles and hour and my car was knocked back eighty-four feet from the impact. My body, upon my return, was crumpled on the floorboard of the backseat.

I don't know how long I'd been gone. My forehead was down to bare skull. From the hairline down to my left eyebrow there was nothing left. It must have been a long time because the layer of blood that soaked my shirt has already dried and caked on my cheeks.

I got out on my own volition. The driver of the other car stumbled towards me. I leaned against the remains of my vehicle. I don't know how long I was there. Time had no reference point. The ambulance driver guided me onto the gurney. I looked up and saw all these people standing around. I didn't know who they were and had no idea what on earth was going on.

The shock wore off on the way to the hospital and I became deeply in touch with my body. The most physical pain I've ever experienced came when the nurse poured sterile water on my forehead. I held the metal bars on the side of the bed as she lightly poured. The pain was so great that I bent the metal bars towards me. The only way to describe the physical sensation is to liken it to slicing a wrist and sticking it in rubbing alcohol. That night I was unable to receive any pain medication because I had a head injury. They woke me every hour on the hour to make sure I had not slipped into a coma. I spent the night asleep and awake, integrating the surreal and the real.

Incredibly, the only apparent damage was the loss of a forehead. The impact didn't crack the skull. They initially thought the severing of all my muscle and skin would have done irreparable damage to my nerves and I might lose the ability to use the right side of my face. They did tests to see if there was any brain damage. They searched for possible neck or spinal injury – nothing was detected.

The only problem was putting the forehead back. They found part of my eyebrow on the backside of my head. The first operation left me with over two hundred stitches. After a couple of more operations I was as good as new. Actually, I still carry a line of scars barely noticeable to most, but they will always look like a neon sign to me. Maybe it's because of where it took me and what was left behind more than my physical vanity. That night, March 3, 1976, was a turning point, to put it mildly. For the next year I spent my interior journey assimilating spirit and body.

To Speak the Unspeakable

The only way I knew to place context to the experience was to fall back on the God of my Fathers. At twenty-one I eased back into Christianity. As I searched spirit looking for words, and found none, I took Christianity's words.

My father's father was a Southern Baptist minister. He was a kind, gentle, deeply in touch with Spirit. He lived in simplistic comfort with who he was and where his feet touched the ground. He was a small town pastor in the backwaters of rural Texas at the time of his death. His baritone laugh vibrated to his core. His silence was dense with peace. He walked too slow, drove too fast and sang hymns too loud. He died in my more tumultuous years and I never really got to sit deeply next to him, but his silhouette still shrouds a tender part of me.

My father's faith took him to do battle with giants. His energy and persistence in social justice were fueled by his unwavering belief in Christ. His journey has taken him around the world to world leaders, movers and shakers. Somewhere between the two I decided to follow the faith of my father. I changed my major to religion, entered a Baptist college, went on to a Baptist seminary and struck out on an impossible task – to describe the indescribable. So, I put my all in an unconscious effort to *fit the Word into words*. Looking back I can see how much of it was to find grounding, a place to stand. I slotted my twenty-three years of life into a pre-packaged belief like a round peg in a square hole.

And when Matt was born, the package broke. It took great effort to pull the pieces back into the box, but it never really fitted the same. I convinced Lydia that a move would do us a world of good. We moved from California to Colorado and from Southern Baptist to the Disciples of Christ, a more moderate denomination.

It was the Disciples of Christ minister in Colorado that asked for my resignation when we found out my family was infected with HIV. In the initial meeting with him he asked for my resignation. I said I wasn't resigning. Our insurance was tied to that particular church and not the denomination. I had three members of my family stricken with catastrophic illnesses. If I had left the church, we would be unable to find insurance with a private carrier.

The next Sunday morning during the Sunday school hour I met him on the stairway. He asked me to join him in his office. The chairman and vice-chair were waiting. We had a discussion about how tragic it all was and then I was told I was not being asked to resign. I was given a leave of absence with two months' salary starting immediately. Sounded a lot like a resignation to me.

Where were we going to find insurance for three people with catastrophic pre-existing conditions? Who would hire me?
It was Phil Strickland, the head of the Texas Baptists Christian Life Commission, who gave me a job.

Phil was a lawyer by education, an ethicist by trade. His heart beats for the disenfranchised. I entered his office for the interview, disheveled by my experience in Colorado and the plight of my wife and children. There are a few bits of the conversation I remember, but the lasting imprint of our first meeting is his soft serenity. Sometimes in a life lived in deserts the oasis is real and not a mirage. This man was real.

Phil and I spoke for quite a while. Then at the end of our conversation he said, "I want you to come here. Even if none of this had happened, I would want to work with you." No one ever worked for Phil. But I never met anyone there that didn't work alongside him. Then he said, "There's one more thing I have to do. When we bring someone on board here we do it as a group. We vote whether someone joins us."

The Christian Life Commission was a department of about ten people. Phil placed my life before these people. The vote was unanimous. In a time when churches were turning us away because they didn't want Matt, ten ordinary people did the extraordinary.

Coming from another denomination, I had to rejoin the Baptists by joining a Baptist Church. The rejection of Matt, Bryan's fading life, Lydia's state of exhaustion and the church's response to HIV left me angry and I was in no mood to join a Baptist church. In fact, the very church that I was able to quietly join was the church that quietly voted for Matt not to be invited. But I had to join because Lydia, Matt and Bryan's health insurance through the Texas Baptists depended on it.

My anger came from an ideal, an expectation that Christianity was what it claimed to be. I wasn't totally naïve. I'd worked in enough churches to see the business side of life. But the blatant rejection of a family because it might drive the ones with money away was a bit much.

I went alone to various churches, various denominations and fellowships looking for some vocabulary, voice and words that would help me understand what was happening to us.

But what kept me within the context of Christianity for as long as I stayed were the people of the Christian Life Commission. Phil and the crew lived an authenticity and a love that was undeniably real, compassionate and woven in true spirit. They never tried to sew the shreds of my life back together. They simply held a space where I was able to day in and day out collect my remains, bring them into the office and place them next to me in my little corner.

Cloistered Sorrow

It is unnatural to be dishonest. We had never had to live like that before. We showed Matt our sorrow for Bryan, but we were always on guard. We calculated every conversation, every gesture, because we knew Matt would likely follow the same path. We hid our exhaustion. We disguised our anguish. We tempered our sadness.

And when night fell, Lydia and I would take to our respective corners until the bell rang and we entered the ring again. Day in and day out, we did battle to create normalcy.

I was not ready for what Bryan's death would do to us. It would seem that when a child dies it would draw the parents closer together. I didn't need to read the studies to know this isn't always the case.

In stress there was a natural tendency for me to slide into whatever mechanism of survival I learned from my childhood. A friend once said, "I don't know who I am, so it's real easy for me to be who I was." *No matter how far I thought I had come, I was left with where I had been.*

My childhood was not the easiest of times and my response was to create little dens for myself where I felt safe. Enclosure comforted me. My family laughed at me because they would frequently find me in my closet, under the bed, or in small places that held what I couldn't. I even set up my entire room at the age of fourteen in my closet, a long, thin cabinet that had a bedroll to sleep on and a little table at my head with candles and a flashlight. The joke was that I just didn't want to clean my room. I wasn't laughing, and it wasn't a joke.

When Bryan died I enclosed again.

Lydia had her own survival mechanisms. She faced each day with resolve. Her blessing was her curse. She had the capacity to endure anything without buckling. She stoically met each day, but the stoicism encased as much as it protected. And in reality, she was more fragile than anyone knew, even me.

At Bryan's funeral, after the eulogy, people mingled. I kept one eye on Matt and spoke to the ones that did their best to find words. Lydia, in her usual graciousness and cool composure, shook hands and said nice things to fill the silence. I wandered off from her in search of Matt. A few minutes later she walked up to me, wrapped her arm under mine and under her breath said, "Don't you ever leave me like that again."

I was shocked. I'd known this woman since I was eleven years old. We had been married for eight years at that time. She was crumbling inside and yet I'd missed the signs. She fooled everyone including me.

Who Suffers? Who Decides?

It was not long after Bryan's funeral when the first of our many conversations about her and Matt's death took place. I remember the street we were on when she first told me. We were on the access road off the highway, heading for my parents' house to pick up Matt. She was calm, even peaceful. She said, "There is something I need to tell you. I've decided that I am never going into the hospital. When I feel like I'm close to the end I'm going to kill myself."

The car eased to a halt three cars back from the red light. I looked at her and nodded. I understood. If I had to endure the death Bryan had just experienced, I would do the same thing.

She went on to say, "And if Matt is in the same condition, I'm going to take him with me."

The light changed. I felt my stomach knot. "What do you mean?"

Her voice was without emotion, but gentle. "I'm not going to let Matt suffer. I will take him with me."

I didn't say anything more. I was unable to digest the magnitude of what Lydia said. Lydia never, never made idle threats. She was not prone to emotionalism or irrationality. I knew she had thought about this for a long time. It took me several days to think through the questions and ramifications of Lydia's decision. The second conversation was in our living room after Matt was asleep. It focused on Matt and her definition of suffering. I asked her, "What is your criteria for taking Matt's life? What suffering? Physically? Socially? Mentally? Is it if he gets dementia? Or if he can't walk?"

She said, "I haven't decided. I'm just not going to let him suffer."

"Lydia, how can you decide the suffering of another?"

"I know suffering. And I'm not going to let my child suffer."

"How do you plan on killing him?" I asked.

"I'm not going to tell you."

She wasn't cold or cruel, which scared me more. Lydia was serious.

"Why won't you tell me?"

She said, "Two reasons. Because it will make you an accomplice. And you might try to stop me."

"Lydia, you have every right to take your own life, but you have no right to take Matt's. You're telling me that you have this criterion for killing him, but you're not going to tell me what it is. You have the way you're going to kill him and you won't tell me how. You can't do this. I have no idea if your idea of his suffering is physical or some other way. What if people find out he's got HIV and they burn our house? Are you going to kill him then?"

She withdrew into silence.

I said, "What if you're sicker than he is, and he's not suffering, what will you do?"

"I don't know. I just know I'm not going to let him suffer. And I don't want to talk about it anymore."

Lydia was finished. I had pushed as far as I could go. If I pressed any further it would have only pushed her further away.

The first year anniversary of Bryan's death was February 2, 1987. I was at work that morning. We lived in Fort Worth, but I worked in downtown Dallas, forty miles from home at the CLC. I called Lydia from the office that morning. There was no answer. I waited thirty minutes and called again. No answer. An hour. No answer.

I left work mid-morning. Forty miles west. What was I to find? Thirty-two miles. Are they dead? Twenty-seven miles. I thought of all the ways she would do it. I thought of never seeing Matt. I thought till my brain went numb. Fifteen miles. Nine. Four. I pulled into the driveway. Her car wasn't there. I exhaled and opened the front door. The house was empty. I called my mother. "Have you seen Matt and Lydia?"

My mother said, "They're over here. Lydia's asleep. She was driving and she couldn't make it home. She stopped here instead."

"What's Matt up to?"

"He's watching TV."

We left Lydia's car at my mother and father's. We went home, put Matt to bed and went to bed. Silent and dark we fell asleep one year to the day after our youngest child died.

Staying Meant Leaving

I was told once that there are about four or five sea kayaks a year that drift off from the island of Maui in Hawaii. The kayak gets caught in the current and is swept away. The person in the boat loses their energy and the small boat slowly slides off to sea never to be seen again.

I don't know if that's really true, but I do know what that is like – to find myself adrift, too tired to try for land.

Grief takes no prisoners. It was my first real taste of what loss leaves. My chaos of spirit was a mixture of preparatory loss and the hole left by Bryan's departure. Which tears belonged to which person? Was my lack of energy a product of the sleepless nights I was recovering from, or the sleepless nights that lay ahead?

Lydia insulated herself in medical journals and potential therapies. I wrapped myself in Matt. But holding Matt was as excruciating as it was beautiful. I couldn't see Matt in the present tense. I'd have him in the morning for another day, but every day was one day closer to when he wouldn't wake again.

Before we found out about the HIV, Matt used to get in the car through the driver's side. He would grab hold of the rear view mirror to balance himself. I was forever wiping tiny fingerprints off the mirror.

When we found out, I started leaving the fingerprints. One day those fingerprints would be gone. I wanted to leave. I wanted to stay. I didn't know what I wanted, but I did know what I didn't want. I didn't want to endure another round like we did with Bryan. The past loomed too large to leave the present alone. Matt and I did our normal rounds of playgrounds and videos; always the past whispered what was to come.

In 1987, I moved out of the house. There was no place to go, no money to go there even if there was some place to run. But my grandfather had an old cottage on the lake outside Brownwood, the town where Bryan was buried. I buried myself there.

Lydia and I continued to co-parent Matt. Any decision made concerning his care was made jointly. I had Matt three and half days out of the week and she took care of him the other days.

Being a part-time father was hard on me. I was used to having Matt every day, living and playing in our normal routine. It was hard on Matt. He was only three, his brother had just died and now his parents had split up.

It was hard on Lydia as well. Her energy was low and she was not used to full-time care on the three and half days he was with her. But Lydia and I had drifted too far by then. There is a difference between stillness and stagnation. We could go through pain and sorrow as long as we stayed fluid in our motion. We could endure anything, anything but stagnation.

Lydia and I sat at the kitchen table. Coffee cups rested in front of us. She softly said, "I feel like we're just waiting for me to die. I feel like I'm waiting to die."

She was right. She continued. "Go. I don't want to live like this. I know you're unhappy."

She was right. I looked from my coffee to her. "I can go to the lake house."

"That'd be good. I need a break," she said.

She was right again. My initial turmoil had settled into an underlying anger. The best way to describe it was that I was like a seething volcano; rarely did I erupt, but there was always rumbling and smoke. She didn't have the stamina to live next to that kind of toxicity. And I don't blame her.

Lydia's strength was to say, "Go." And her ability to go on was hallmark Lydia.

There was never any doubt that we would be there for each other and for Matt. We just couldn't be there in the same way. The stagnation was too great. The weight of the present tense froze, locked in tomorrow's yesterdays.

The small cottage by Lake Brownwood had been in the family since I was around nine. The neighbor next door, Buck, was living there when my grandfather bought the place in 1965. His wife had died ten or fifteen years earlier. Buck's body was still strong, but the cancer was slowly eating him away when I moved in next door.

Buck was a bridge to a time past. Like the cottage itself, Buck was part of memory that accumulates, holding the pieces together.

The Test

I decided to get tested again for HIV. It had been several years. Even though I used universal precautions around any blood spill and we used condoms, I wanted to make sure I was still HIV negative. It was like someone who goes to a fortune teller to see the future. I wanted to make sure, to know what the future may hold.

I went to the anonymous test site at the Dallas County Health Department. The aging building stood across the street from Parkland Hospital. I walked in the door feeling like I was wearing a neon sign. People milled around the lower floor. My eyes were glued to the linoleum floor as I took the steps up to the clinic. The waiting room had one other person waiting. We both buried our heads in magazines.

My number was called and I went into the back cubical with the nurse. She sat behind the desk and asked me questions. There weren't a lot of straight men, with a wife and child infected with HIV and with another child that had died a year earlier, banging down the door of the Dallas County Health Department. I was given a number on a piece of paper and I shoved it in my pocket. She pushed her hand into the rubber glove, prepared the needle and slapped a tourniquet on my arm. My blood filled the vial.

In those days, the state of Texas only did the ELISA test, the procedure that was highly sensitive and used mainly for screening blood donations. They did not do the Western Blot, the confirmatory test, unless specifically requested. The ELISA test took two weeks for the results because the Dallas County Health Department sent all the samples to the state lab in Austin.

I went back to Brownwood, a four-hour drive…to wait. There was a heaviness to the drive. Lydia and I had been married for almost nine years. We'd never been separated before. I'd never been separated from Matt. All my life I've spent time alone, but in the circumference of others. I may have wandered to the edge of the circle, but I always rested within relationship.

The ride home wasn't to home at all. It was a house that I played in during summer as a child. Emptiness filled me.

I had created the one scenario I dreaded most – empty aloneness. I'd curl in until it was my turn to have Matt during the week. Then I would unfurl enough to love. It was summer. Matt and I would play in the water just like I played when I was young. We took walks in the rocky back woods. He mainly rested on my shoulders as we explored the little hideouts I had as a child. We had perpetual slumber parties, but only Friday nights' tossing and tumbling was called "rowdy night." We soaked in every moment…and I waited.

I had tested negative in the whirlwind of Colorado. The waiting then was so caught up in the chaos I didn't have time to think. This waiting was different. I had a lot of time on my own to think.

Two weeks was up and I returned to the Dallas County Health Department. The same nurse sat me down. Her countenance was firm, but not grim. She wasted no time once we were settled in our chairs. She said, "Your test results are back. You tested positive for AIDS. I'm sorry."

My body was numb. I left with a pamphlet.

The four-hour drive back to Brownwood was surreal. The main question for me was how did I get here from there? One day I was sitting on the steps of a parsonage with Lydia talking to our child in her womb. I turn around and I'm driving to the only place I have left, completely mystified.

I called Lydia. Whenever Lydia experienced overwhelming news, she grew more calm and controlled. She instinctively practiced the middle way of emotional stability. She said, "Go get the Western Blot. The ELISA is too sensitive and it could be wrong."

I never thought I believed in a punishing God. If the test were wrong, what kind of God would play such a cruel joke?

Sitting alone in the living room of my dead grandfather's lake house — a few miles from the buried casket of my youngest son, one hundred and seventy miles from my wife and three-year-old child, within a body that now had a measured time — I reflected on fate.

I blamed the man that gave the blood. I blamed the blood bank for not screening the blood. I blamed God. I blamed me. The futility of blame was lost on me as I paced the rooms at night. The next week, when I was in Dallas for business, I went back to the County Health Department. The same nurse took the same blood. But this time I would have to wait a month to get the results of the Western Blot.

I waited the month. I spent my days alone. My aunt and uncle were the only people I knew in Brownwood and I rarely saw them by my own accord. I took walks, sat next to the brown water and stared at walls that held my childhood.

I would see Buck from time to time sitting next to his picture window. He stationed himself there so he could see the one lane gravel road in the front of the house. On my walks a wave from his living room would often condemn me to innocuous conversations. We avoided anything deep while he was waiting to die and I was waiting to see if I was going to die.

A month passed. Again, the same nurse sat me down. Her face tried to conceal the bad news. I had inhaled just on the outskirts of Dallas and before I could exhale sitting across from her, she said, "I'm sorry. It appears we have messed up. We are going to have to take another blood sample."

I exhaled. "What happened?"

"I don't know. From what I understand they dropped the vial or something and they couldn't test the sample."

She took more blood. I drove home to wait another month.

I was worn out. My brain had exhausted me and I was drifting further from land like the kayak out to sea. The only ground I could stand on was next to Matt. The days we were apart I paddled against the current as best I could knowing that on Wednesday I'd be safe till Saturday.

It was almost three months since I first entered the health department. I had lost any self-consciousness as I climbed the steps to the waiting room. We sat in her office. She said, "The test results are back. Your Western Blot is positive."

The Western Blot was the definitive kiss of death in 1987. I walked out of the building in an out-of-body experience. By rote I drove four hours back to Brownwood, sinking into a waiting death.

I pulled up in front of the house. Buck waved from his window. I waved back, pretending he was waving just to say hello and walked directly to my front door. I didn't want to talk, listen or think. I lay down on the bed and stared at the ceiling.

For the first time I understood Lydia. I stepped into Lydia's world, the one she woke to every morning. It was different not because life was different, but because death was different. Transformation of the mundane seemed to take place in every movement. City street corners filled with souls rather than people. The planet grew small and intimate. A rock held mountains. A drop of water held an ocean. And love, especially love lost, clothed the seconds that ticked to the beat of time like a meter.

Lydia and I spoke often. She knew that now I knew and she opened a part of her that could not be articulated to others. She was still calm and controlled, but now I could see it wasn't to push me away. It was because what held her together was impossible to articulate. My frustration evolved into a deep admiration for a woman who withstood so much with such dignity and grace. I witnessed how Lydia reflected that place where earth and sky meet.

The Last to Care

I understood why Lydia said she planned to take her own life, for I decided to do the same. But I didn't have her inner fortitude. I was not going to wait till my physicality diminished to a whisper. I was finished, there and then.

I set off from Brownwood on a farewell visit to my past. My most formative years were spent growing up in San Antonio, Texas. I drove the back roads towards San Antonio full of unanswerable questions, self-pity and memories. I just wanted to make sense of something before I died. I drove past the house we lived and the schools I attended. I went to the spot where I had the car accident. I tried to look up some old friends. I found out that one of my best friends, Cecil Martinez, had moved down to Padre Island, a town down at the tip of the border between Texas and Mexico.

Cecil and I were close. We spent a lot of high school together and were roommates in our first year of college. I hadn't seen Cecil in over fourteen years. I figured I'd see him one more time. Besides, I'd never seen Padre Island and that was as good a place to die as anywhere else.

Cecil was still Cecil – warm, friendly, wonderful sense of humor and wise enough not to pretend he understood. We had traveled through some rough experiences growing up. In high school his parents went through a difficult divorce and the insanity in my family was in full swing. We laughed and joked our way through the ups and downs. Cecil's heart was strong enough to break and open enough to find renewal.

South Padre was warm. The sandy beaches rest up against the Gulf of Mexico. Cecil welcomed me with open arms. I shared my story with him that night. I also shared my plan to commit suicide.
Cecil listened, but what could anybody say? He tried, but I was far too gone in my poor pitiful me.

At two in the morning I got behind the wheel of my 1979 Plymouth Charade searching for an available tree to crash into. The small engine whined its way to its top speed of ninety-five miles an hour. The steering wheel shook. The tires bounced on the empty country road. I went into my final diatribe of disappointments. "Nobody loves me. Lydia doesn't love me. My parents don't love me. God doesn't love me."

Then something happened. I had touched a moment of clarity. I said to myself, "F… it. *I* love me." The dreamer caught the dream catcher just in time and I didn't die. I was touched by something within and beyond me. An epiphany descended upon me and the moment suspended. A feeling of warmth moved from within and swept over me.

I found that somewhere in the recesses of me was the capacity to love. Love led me to the decision to live as constructively as I could for as long as I could. I would do what I could to give to life rather than take. It was a fragile truce at best, but I had decided to die when death came, and not a moment earlier.

I pulled the car over to the side of the road and fell asleep. I woke up the next morning and headed back to Brownwood.

"I'm Not Going to Make It."

As I pulled up in front of the cottage, Buck did more than wave this time. He rose painfully from his chair and opened his door. He specifically asked me to come in.

Buck's dining table was cluttered with pill bottles.

He looked fairly fit for his aging years, but the cancer significantly weakened him.

He wanted to talk about life, our shared history, and his wife whom he dearly loved and I lovingly remembered. He periodically rubbed his fingers through his thick white hair and stared off into space. Interspersed in between memories, Buck would say, "I'm not going to make it, Scotty."

I hate the name Scotty because it is the name of my childhood, but Buck had earned the right to call me that. To him I was still a young child he took fishing off his dock, skiing behind his boat and for swims along with his wife.

Many times Buck shook his head and said, "I'm not going to make it."

I wanted to ask, but didn't. I wanted to say, "Buck, what are you trying to make it to?"

The man had lived into his late seventies. He had had a full life. I was thirty and facing death, too. I would soon have pill bottles scattered on my table just like him.

He shook his head again. "I'm just not going to make it."

That weekend Matt came to stay as usual. We were still asleep that morning when the phone rang. It was my aunt. She said, "Don't let Matt go outside. Buck has hung himself on the water tower."

The silver water tower sat directly across from our cottage. A metal ladder was bolted next to the tall cylinder. Buck, using the last of his strength, had climbed up to the second tier. He wrapped a rope around the large bar, wrapped the other end of the rope around his neck, and jumped.

Buck wasn't able to wait for the stillness of night and for death to come in his sleep. God wasn't coming. Buck had to go find God instead.

Not too many came to see Buck in his last days, but his lodge brothers were there for the funeral. His son said that he'd taken the shotgun out of Buck's house for fear that something like this would happen.

When I returned from the funeral the metal ladder had been sawn off just out of arm's reach.

Somebody Else's Life

About a quarter of a mile from the cottage lays the dam. Rock cut into boulders, artificially placed to keep the water from flowing.

I walked those rocks barefoot in the heat of summer. I slowly set my feet on the uneven surface, measuring my movements by centimeters.

My toes touched rock and my racing mind calmed. The uneven surface brought me balance of mind and body. It brought me into the present tense. And once I was able to sit in the present I was able to reflect on what to do next.

Lydia and I decided to give it another try. Of all the gifts I received in this period of my life, one stands out. It was the freedom from guilt. I had lived with enormous survivor's guilt. Why were they being taken and not I? We now stood under the same light in the same journey. I said to Lydia in discussing our reunion, "If anyone can understand what we are going through it would be each other." The road narrowed enough for both of us to fit.

My commitment on Padre Island to give back to life for as long as life was to be, led me to the Dallas Interfaith Conference on AIDS. It was where I met Father Ted. Father Ted was an Episcopal priest, a sharp man with a hide thick enough to do the right thing. He knew how to maneuver through the ecclesiastical shark-infested waters. He had started a ministry for people with HIV in his parish and wanted to expand the care to others. This conference was the beginning of a collective religious response to the epidemic, a much needed move by 1987.

I told Ted my story. I volunteered to do pastoral counseling to anyone in need. If anyone could understand what he or she was enduring it was I.

Ted worked closely with the Dallas County Health Department and the anonymous test site where I was tested. He told my story there. Like I mentioned earlier, the health department had not yet seen a lot of fathers with a wife and child living with HIV and another child recently deceased. Actually, they had seen none at that stage. The nurse that tested me all those many times happened to be at the meeting. She approached Ted after he shared my profile to the group and said to him, "This has got to be the same person. We gave him the wrong results."

Ted called me. His voice was light and exploding at the same time. He said, "You're negative."

I sat at my desk at the Baptist General Convention of Texas stunned. I listened to Ted explain what had happened.

What are the odds that an anonymous test site in a city of millions would find me? I was seconds from my death in that car. I thought months, perhaps a year, from death with the infection. And in one phone call I was told it was not real, just part of the dream.

I went to Janet, Matt's pediatrician, and got tested again. Negative.

Later I worked closely with the Dallas County Health Department and the director. In one informal meeting with the doctor I asked him, "Was it a false positive or did I get somebody else's result?" It turns out it was somebody else's. For three months I thought I was going to die; and for a period of time this person thought he was going to live.

No Different At All

Father Ted and Buck Buckingham, the first director of AIDS ARMS, managed to bring me on as the coordinator of the AIDS Interfaith Network. AIDS ARMS was, and is, a network of service providers for HIV patients and their families. AIDS Interfaith was created to provide supportive and confidential spiritual care for patients as well as educate local religious bodies of all faiths about HIV. One of the tasks in which I participated was going to homes of people with HIV. I listened to their stories, and when they requested a community congruent with their beliefs, I approached the head of a like-minded local institution. I was a guard at the gate of a fragile person and hopefully a healing place of spirit.

I went to a young man's house. He was still healthy, recently diagnosed. He desperately wanted to make me a sandwich. He took great care in his preparation. A grilled cheese sandwich was his way to leap the chasm between HIV and everything else.

"You can't get AIDS through the handling of food," he said as he flipped the sandwich on the other side.

I sat at his table watching him. "No," I said, "you can't." He nodded and kept his eyes on the smoldering pan. "I was at the grocery store today. I stood in this line. I knew they were all looking at me. I knew they knew. Like they could see I had AIDS. I was really scared."

He looked at me with an exhausted half smile. "I really knew they didn't know, but it felt like it."

His shoulders lowered as he looked into my eyes. I nodded again, but let the silence still his racing spirit. He lowered his eyes again to the grill. "I feel so dirty. I'm so ashamed."

"Of what?" I asked. "Ashamed of love?"

He searched my expression to see if I was making a joke. "What do you mean?"

"We are all reaching for love. I assume you became infected through sex. What is sex but an attempt on one level or another to feel and experience love."

It took me over three years to work through my anger and blame. In my mind we were "innocent." We didn't do anything. And if we didn't do anything someone must have. My anger focused on the gay community, a natural target for a Southern Baptist minister. I thought back to the protest in the early eighties in San Francisco when the health department targeted some of the bathhouses. Anger and blame places people and places into categories of them and us. Lydia and I had been faithful. Us/Them.

Fortunately, I moved past the illusion of separation into the common denominator. At the first Interfaith Network Conference in Dallas I told Father Ted that I was still working through my emotions around the gay community. He introduced me to a man whose partner had just died.

The man was in his late fifties. The lines under his eyes were deep and his cheeks hung flaccidly on the curve of his jaw. His straight brown hair was peppered with gray. In a strong, slow Texas accent he spoke of the love he had for his partner of sixteen years.

I only remember snippets of the conversation; two in particular come to mind. What I remember most were his eyes. These were my eyes. I saw the same expression, the same weight of sorrow every morning when I looked in the mirror. His voice was my voice. I echoed the same weariness. His love was my love. He tenderly spoke of the one he loved and it was the same love I loved Lydia.

He said, "Take lots of pictures." That was his only advice to me in that one and only conversation. Take lots of pictures.

The other part of the conversation that leaned my path into healing was when I said to him, "I still have a lot of anger with the gay community."

He, in a soft, gentle voice, asked, "How do you know the guy that gave your wife the blood was gay?"

Anger and blame blinds. He was right. I began thinking of the man I never knew, the one that gave blood. Was it because he felt it was his civic duty to give to life and the blood mobile came tooling up to his work place asking for donations? Was he a junkie in need of cash? Who was this man?

I looked at the man sitting across the table from me. The man that was me. What would I say to this man if he was the one that gave the blood that the blood bank gave Lydia? This soft, gentle man that carried no malice, no sediments of hatred, no self-pity. He was a kind man, with my eyes, my voice, my love.

The grilled cheese sandwich was a bit on the burned side. He didn't know I ate sandwiches made by someone with HIV all the time. For Lydia and I agreed that as long as we could keep Matt's life as close to normal as possible, we would live in secret. I picked up the simple slice of cheese melted between two white pieces of bread. He watched as I took a bite. The underlying panic that vibrated through him like a low fever eased. His face relaxed. His body sank into the chair. He said, "I'm no different from anybody else."

"No," I said. "No different at all."

Bryan's House

It was in my capacity as the AIDS Interfaith coordinator that I met Lynn. She was moving closer to the final stages of AIDS by the time we met. Her husband and two young children were HIV-negative. Lydia met often with Lynn. They shared their stories and a common language.

We had already moved to Dallas from Fort Worth. It was nearer to the Baptist office and the AIDS Interfaith Network. More importantly, we wanted to settle Matt into a place more permanent before we faced the gauntlet of securing him passage in the public school system.

Dr. Janet Squires and her family had moved to Dallas as well. She became the head of the HIV care unit at Children's Medical Center.

Lynn's husband did what he could, but a laborer must labor in order to eat. The children were old enough to know and too young to care for themselves. Lynn was Lydia's inspiration for a house to help families with HIV.

Lydia's sole mission became the creation of the house. She joined forces with another woman in the community, Stephanie Held. They worked at fundraising, grant writing, networking and providing a place for the children to come. Janet joined in the fray as well.

Lynn became sicker. The house was still in the planning and

foundational stage when one day Lydia and I went to the hospital to see Lynn. She was emaciated; an air tube stretched under her nose; an IV bottle loomed above her. She turned to Lydia. "The doctor said I'm really sick and I'm going to die. I don't feel that bad. Do you think I look that bad?"

Lydia gracefully said, "Well Lynn, you are pretty sick."

Lynn's eyes had already turned inward by that stage. The look was there.

I had seen the look before. It became commonplace in the land between life and death – the vacuous look that comes when someone sees more of what's coming than what's been, or what appears to be. Those eyes used to disturb me. I would sit watching the emptying of the eyes and feel the distance grow wider. But I came to a place of peace with the vacant stare. I started to see it as not an emptying, but a refocusing. The look became a promise, a turn of the spirit to gaze upon another place, deep inside. It was no longer a leaving of this world, but an entering into another. Lynn's eyes did not disturb me.

She looked at me and I shrugged my shoulders, "Who knows?"

Lynn scratched her matted hair. "Yeah, who knows?"

Lynn died the next day.

Lydia wasn't at the children's house board meeting when the name for the house was discussed. I understand that it was Janet who suggested the name be Bryan's House, after one of the first children in the area to die from AIDS. I think Lydia was touched by the gesture, but the only thing she ever said to me concerning the name was "That's nice."

Lydia never lost focus on what the house was there to do and for whom. She wanted to leave something meaningful behind, something that made sense out of the senselessness we faced daily. There was never any doubt that Lydia's myopic effort to bring this house into fruition was to ease the path of families like Lynn's. She didn't care all that much about leaving behind a name; but she did leave an indelible trace of spirit in a house that still cares for children today.

Lydia thought after the initial diagnosis that she'd never be able to use her nursing skills again, but Janet brought Lydia to work at the HIV clinic. She sat with mothers whose children were sick, some close to death. She, at times, nursed those far less sick than she was, but rarely did she share her plight with the patients she cared for. It was difficult enough for the ones close to Lydia to penetrate very deep into her world. But for the patients and their caregivers, Lydia was a professional. AZT and sheer grit gave Lydia more strength. AZT was definitely no cure-all. Its toxic side effects had to be weighed against the benefits; but without AZT, the first medical intervention for HIV, Lydia would have died much earlier. She described herself as Matt's guinea pig, the test case. Ultimately Matt went on the AZT as well.

Teachers and Students, Students and Teachers

The moment of truth was at hand. Matt was old enough for school. Across the country there was a time of reckoning with school districts coming to grips with HIV-infected children. Lydia said, "Someday the truth will catch up with the facts."

The school district policy was for the child to have a medical examination and a confidential interview with the top school officials to determine whether the child was a risk to other children. Janet and three school officials met with Lydia and me. Matt received the go ahead to attend, but there was a complication. Matt's birth date of October left him one month late of a mandatory attendance in the school we were assigned. The school was full and he would have to go to a neighboring school.

Lydia went to enroll Matt. We thought it was going to be just a mere formality and everything had been set, so I didn't go. The district policy was that only the principal, teacher and school nurse were to know of a child's HIV status. Lydia clearly recognized that the principal was not informed.

Since we had decided from the first days that an adult would know and be present with Matt, she told the principal. The principal called in the kindergarten teacher and Lydia talked to her as well. The principal said that she didn't want Matt in the school. The teacher also said she wouldn't teach Matt. Both refused to let Matt enroll.

Lydia was devastated, again. The rejection of Matt was her greatest fear and here it was. We had gone through all the proper channels and this was the outcome. Everyone was left with an impassable situation. The school district scrambled to solve the "problem." Our confidentiality teetered on finding someone to accept our child and hold dear our secret.

Father Ted shared our plight in a prayer meeting at his parish and asked for prayer. Ruth, a parishioner, approached him after the meeting. She was the principal of an inner city school. She said she would talk to the kindergarten teacher and see if Matt could enter there. Without hesitation Matt was invited to attend their school.

Joyce, his brand new kindergarten teacher, perpetually glowed. She was short and her round black cheeks stretched into a beautiful smile when Matt entered the room. Lydia and I had already met her and her calm, warm spirit kindled confidence in us both. She didn't seem the type to get ruffled, a valuable quality when at the helm of eleven or so five-year-olds.

Joyce did something very special the first day Matt entered the room. Joyce didn't treat Matt special. He was the only white child in the class, but Joyce didn't see color. He was the only kid with HIV, but Joyce's gentleness saw a child full of life, just like the rest of her class. In a world where Lydia and I felt we no longer fit, and where Matt was an outsider as well, Joyce treated us like we were just two parents of one of her students. She taught more than just our child that year.

I picked Matt up from school on most days. This particular day it was Martin Luther King's birthday. Matt leapt into the car and with wide eyes and utter amazement he said, "Did you know somebody shot Arthur Luther King?"

I matched his wide eyes. "What! They shot his brother, too?"

Matt said, "Yeah! Why would they do that?"

The conversation turned to those who stand up for what is right, those that go against the current. We talked in general terms, but as we talked on the way home, I thought of Joyce.

Matt scurried into the house to tell Lydia about Martin Luther King like it was just on the morning news. I dropped his backpack on the couch, sat down as he went into great detail to Lydia about his day, and I felt something very special. For a brief moment I felt absolutely normal.

The next year Matt was to attend his required school. Again we met with the principal, teacher and school nurse. For some unknown reason, the school secretary attended as well. This time I was there.

Larry, the principal, greeted us at the door. He was a round man, kind and easy going. Marion was to be Matt's teacher. Larry spoke of the complications we faced.

The school had a mixture of highly affluent kids and other children on the edge of poverty. Fear has no economic borders and some of our discussion focused on what would happen if Matt's confidentiality was broken.

The secretary was apparently a pessimist by nature. She said, "You're going to regret the day you enrolled your child in Lakewood Elementary." Larry tempered her "cheery" outlook with words of comfort. Fortunately, Larry was a man to be believed. We could feel his integrity as well as his warmth. We felt from our first meeting with Larry that he would protect Matt and stand up against anyone that tried to deny Matt a place in his school.

Marion, the teacher, was a strong woman, intelligent and articulate. She was the kind of person that spoke her mind. Her words were crisp, on the edge of forcefulness. She said she was willing to teach Matt, but she wanted to be tested for HIV before the school year in case she became infected. This request was not for fear of Matt. It was her fear of a lack of support from the school district. Still, Lydia and I, burned in the past, were skeptical of how she would treat Matt.

We needn't have worried. Matt worked his magic on her, and before the end of the year Marion had offered to baby-sit for us. In a time of living in secret and never leaving Matt with someone that didn't *know*, we felt like we had won the lottery.

She and Matt had the same kind of humor, wicked and in abundance. The cartoon, *Ninja Turtles*, had just hit the screen. The main characters' names were Donatello, Michelangelo, Raphael and Leonardo. Matt would come to class and tell Marion all about these turtles. Marion decided to show the other teachers what kind of students she had. She prepped Matt before she took him into the teacher's lounge and said, "Matt, give us the names of four famous Renaissance painters."

Matt, her unwitting accomplice, reeled them off: "Donatello, Michelangelo, Raphael, and Leonardo." They both had a good laugh and made a shared memory that day.

The secretary's ominous warning plagued me for years. Every morning when I dropped Matt off at school I was shadowed by the question: What if they find out? What will they do to Matt?

Lydia and I went to PTA meetings and pretended to be normal. Lydia would be so sick some PTA nights that she could barely manage the walk from the car to the auditorium. However, she always managed to transform completely into just another mother with just another child when we entered. She was not going to give anyone room to question how she was. If they found out about her, they would find out about Matt, and that was out of the question.

Lydia and I were always on the lookout for Matt's socialization. I was out of town the day of enrollment in a father/son group for six-year-olds so Lydia went to the initial meeting of the fathers. She was the only mother in the group, but she enrolled us into the YMCA program.

It was ideal for us. I could always be with Matt on the campouts and day excursions and he could be with other kids. We'd swim together, ride horses and shoot bows and arrows. There were five fathers, five sons in our group. Every meeting or campout I wondered, what if they knew? What will happen when they find out?

Matt met a boy named Zack in a YMCA swim class when he was five. Zack had black hair, a sense of humor like Matt's and a tender heart.

Zack invited Matt to a sleepover. Lydia and I knew this day would come. We had to talk to Zack's parents and tell them if Matt was to be out without us.

Kurt and Barbara met us at their door. Our worst fear wasn't that we tell them and they might say no. Our greatest fear was that they might tell everyone and then every child and parent might turn on us and ostracize Matt. It was a great risk. But the more we talked to them the more comfortable we became. Lydia and I looked at each other and decided to take the chance. They listened and empathized. Then they said they would speak to their pediatrician. We offered to let them talk to Janet. They also reassured us that our conversation would not leave the room.

The next day Zack called Matt and asked him to spend the night. Zack became Matt's best friend. Zack's little sister, Alison, became like a little sister, mutually tormented by both Zack and Matt. And Kurt and Barbara opened their home to him.

Matt, Zack and I had a special game when Zack spent the night at our house. We would turn off all the lights and play a version of "hide and seek" with a fringe element of "tag, you're it." Mayhem swept the house as we laughed, bumped into chairs and stealthed through the house.

Every time Zack entered the house a touch of normalcy descended. The enclosure we experienced disintegrated when someone outside our pain entered our world. It was more than a child coming to play with our son. It was an inclusion into a life no longer available to us, a normalcy that we remembered and could at least stand next to in what seemed to be a parallel universe.

The Dream within the Dream

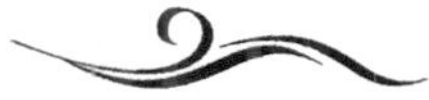

Lydia and I had been waiting to tell Matt about his HIV status for five years. Matt was now seven. For five years Lydia and I had been in perpetual preparation for this conversation. Every time he physically couldn't keep up with the other kids we handled it as if it was no big deal. We tried to make it a game when he went for his monthly IV treatments. After they had stuck a needle in him and poured the medicine in for an hour and half, we went to the toy store to get a special prize and made it a celebration. We had worked hard to make the abnormal normal. We knew that every day, every event led to this day when he would put it all together.

We had already talked to Kurt and Barbara about preparing Zack for Matt's news. Matt knew something was different about him. Other children didn't go to the hospital once a month for intravenous treatments of gamma globulin. Matt wasn't growing like the other children. Zack shot up in height, but Matt remained short and stocky in his early years.

Lydia and I felt that Matt always knew there was something he didn't know. He was very intuitive from his earliest days.

Lydia and I had planned everything.

We had children's books on HIV. We had Zack waiting for a call. We had several meetings with his therapist to discuss all the ramifications and she was waiting in the wings to meet with him. We planned what we were going to say and when.

It was Friday afternoon after school. We wanted it to be right before rowdy night so Matt and I would have time to talk it over. Another plus was it was the beginning of the weekend and he would have a few days to process the information before sitting in a classroom of his friends.

Everything was to be put out in the open. That night we were going to tell our child not only that he had HIV, but we were ready to speak frankly to him about Bryan and how Bryan died if he asked. Lydia was also going to tell him she was infected and how.

This was the hardest topic for Lydia because it forced her to face the inevitability of her leaving Matt. It was apparent by then that her body was breaking down and he was relatively stable. We knew we had the task of preparing Matt for Lydia's death.

Lydia's voice was a manufactured calmness. She tried to sound ordinary, but Matt knew.

She said, "Matt, we need to talk to you about something."

Matt was in the living room on the couch. He heard something in her voice that made him stop and focus his attention on her.

She said, "You have a special condition. You've probably wondered why we take you to the hospital every month for treatments."

His voice was reserved. "Yeah."

Lydia went on. She spoke of the HIV and how he was infected. She told him she had it, too. We told him how she got it and what we were doing medically to try to make it better for both of them. We didn't mention Bryan that Friday afternoon and Matt didn't ask.

Matt knew it was something serious, but didn't want to know anymore. When we asked him if he had any questions he said no.

We asked him again. "Are you sure you don't have any questions?"

Matt became angry. He said, "NO! I want to have rowdy now. Come on, Papa."

Lydia and I looked at each other. Matt was definitely his mother's child. When a conversation was over, it was over.

I didn't mention the HIV during rowdy. Matt definitely didn't bring it up. We had pretended for so long and without realizing it, we had taught our child how to pretend, too.

That night I had a dream. Matt and I were in an empty room. We sat on the floor facing a screen that covered the entire wall. There was a Presence in the room, not a tangible presence, just a sense of another joining us. Matt and I snuggled next to each other and we watched various lives pass by on a large projector like a movie. We watched six lives in detail. I said, "Matt, remember when you were this…?"

"Yeah, Papa."

Another life crossed the screen and I said, "Matt, remember when I was this and you were that?"

"Yeah, Papa, I remember."

The dream changed and Matt and I were walking in heaven. Heaven wasn't a place. It was a state of being. There was serenity and peace, but nothing seen or unseen. It wasn't like my near-death experience in its external manifestation, but it was the same state of being.

Matt and I strolled the nebulous condition looking around. I said, "See Matt, we're still going to know each other here. We're still going to be together."

Matt said, "Yeah, Papa, this is nice."

I woke from the dream into the other dream. Matt was still asleep. I looked at the soul that was my child, reliving the dream.

I loved watching Matt sleep. Any parent will testify that their child's sleeping state is filled with a peaceful radiance. I would often go into Matt's room and watch him dream.

Darkness is much clearer in the deepness of night. Darkness does not disturb me. It reminds me to sink into my stillness. Whenever I step into a dark moment I rest in motionlessness to let my eyes adjust. It is amazing what illuminations live in darkness. Thoughts sink into thought like sound turning to whisper, turning to silence. Silence turns into a soundless language carried softly by the dark.

I used to be scared of the dark as a child. I slept with a light on. *Dreams clinging to an artificial nightlight.* But as I grew, my heart stopped racing in one place and stillness moved me further into the soft abyss where the black pearl hangs, where shadows live and breathe, whispering.

I fell back asleep next to Matt, out of the shadow into a dreamless sleep. Morning woke us both. I made him breakfast and we watched Saturday morning cartoons. I wanted to tell him about the dream, but not this morning.

Lydia wasn't there that morning when I asked him again. "Matt, are you sure you don't have any questions at all about the HIV. That's some pretty heavy duty stuff and I just want to make sure you understand."

Again he said, "No!"

I took another run. "Please, Matt. I need to know you know what's going on. Isn't there any question at all?"

There was a hint of frustration like he just wanted me to get off his back. Matt asked, "Can you die from this?"

I softly said, "Yes, Matt, you can die from this."

The frustration was gone. His voice became soft and subdued. "How?"

"Would you like to read this book?" I pulled out the book on HIV written for children. The brightly colored pictures and simple words describe how a virus works. It didn't go into its ultimate work, but Matt knew.

He asked, "Did Bryan die of HIV?"

"Yes, Bryan died of HIV."

He wanted to know in more detail how he got it. I told him about the complications at his birth. I told him about the blood bank. How they didn't screen the blood or take the precautions to do other tests that would have eliminated the potential carrier from donating the blood. He wanted to know about the donor. Like everyone else, Matt tried to make sense of it all by trying to figure out who or why, but the underlying element of the question of who or why is always who is to blame. I told him the donor didn't know. It wasn't his fault. He was just trying to do the right thing. We talked more about the blood bank. How do you talk to a seven-year-old about the corporate greed and irresponsibility? Later, I asked Matt if he wanted to draw a picture to show me what he was feeling. He jumped at the chance. He called to me from the other room and said, "How do you spell son of a bitch?"

"Why?"

"I'm drawing a picture of the man at the blood bank," he said as he held up the picture.

I said, "S-o-n-o-f-a-b-i-t-c-h."

Matt and I went on a walk later that morning. He needed to have a physical outlet as well as emotional expression. He asked all sorts of questions on our walk. He unloaded everything that he knew, but didn't know. I unloaded everything I'd held for years waiting for that day.

We talked about whom he wanted to tell, which friends were safe and who might be unkind and misunderstand. I was amazed at Matt's replies as we went through the list. Of course he wanted to tell Zack. The remarkable part of the rest of the list was just how congruent our assessments of who would probably be safe and who wouldn't. I'd say a name and Matt would either say yes or no. At seven years old Matt was a quick read of people.

I acted like the whole conversation was just a run of the mill chat, as if we were talking about the laws of gravity, but I was deeply relieved. Now Matt and I could speak without hiding. The texture of our journey together deepened that day. More than information fitted into place. Matt and I found a resting place for the truth. As difficult as it was, it was infinitely easier than holding something from him.

Yet, it wasn't time to tell him of the dream, the lives or the Presence. The dream needed time to settle. But it was the dream that sustained my calmness. This dream within the dream was to foreshadow other dreams, other moments, and otherness in and of itself.

Matt went over to Zack's that afternoon. I'll never know what they talked about or what Zack said, but Matt came home in peace.

The next day I picked up Matt at the summer day care. Barbara was there, waiting for Zack. I said, "Barbara, thank you so much for all you are doing for Matt."

She said, "It's the least we could do."

I said, "No, Barbara, it's the most you could do."

Isolation at 20,000 Feet

Lydia, Matt and I carefully chose the ones to tell. Matt did not want to tell the entire school. He preferred to just tell close friends. Lydia and I paved the way by preparing the parents just like we did with Kurt and Barbara. Each peek over the edge of uncertainty was measured with trepidation. If that hurdle was passed, there was still no guarantee the seven-year-old friend would not tell the whole school and parents unknown to us would rise in protest. The anxiety of holding a secret was not much different from the anxiety of a shared secret.

Lydia and I agreed not to share our plight in public for as long as we could. If the entire school caught wind of Matt's condition then we would take the offensive. We would set it all out and put the spotlight on our situation as strongly as we could. The best defense we believed was a strong offense. We were keenly aware of what happened to Ryan White, a young teenager in Indiana. When the truth came out, his community turned him away and it was a very painful rejection. We set out a strategy of preparing leaders to lead, which had not happened in Ryan's community. The right people in key positions did not take the lead and speak out. With our work in the HIV community, we were able to quietly move in circles that would be the first voices to speak if parents found out. I met with the mayor, who graciously agreed to support Matt if it came out. I met with government representatives on state and federal levels, voices strong enough to be heard. The school board was poised to speak. We were ready.

Several times through our work or the grapevine, a newspaper reporter would catch wind of the story. Each and every time the reporter agreed not to print it. Good people doing good things. The reporters would have had a fleeting story that would have changed our entire lives and I am deeply grateful for the integrity of the news people that crossed our path.

But it became increasingly difficult to maintain silence. I worked mainly with Baptist churches in HIV education, but I also spoke in synagogues and in other religious communities. I encountered a wide variety of responses.

The conservative churches were a lesson in contrasts. There were people advocating quarantining people with HIV. They always started out by saying, "How do we know it is not more infectious? How can we trust the health officials? I think we should…."

Then, there were the ones sitting in the crowd who held broken hearts. They held the shadow of a child or spouse, a grandmother or lover, a husband or brother in their eyes.

I told Lydia, "I feel like a boxer that enters the ring with his hands tied behind his back." It wore me thin and left me weary, but Lydia was adamant that it wasn't time to share our story.

In 1988, I was appointed to the Texas Legislative Task Force on AIDS. The task force was assigned to travel the state and provide legislative recommendations for Texas.

The first meeting was in Houston. There was a large crowd of print reporters and cameras at the gathering. The panel members were asked to introduce themselves and what they brought to the process. I was absolutely terrified. What if someone asked about Matt? His entire school situation and personal life hung precariously in the room. I muttered something about being with the Texas Baptist Christian Life

Commission and volunteer coordinator of the Dallas AIDS Interfaith Network. The façade held and the day ended.

The commuter flight from Houston to Dallas takes a little over an hour. Business people with Armani and Gucci costumes packed the flight. My costume consisted of Hush Puppy shoes and a K-Mart "blue light special" sports coat tossed over the seat next to me. I had learned from experience not to take my tie off because I would somehow forget it or destroy it, so the knot was loose and dangled like a noose. Buttoned long sleeve shirts feel like handcuffs to me so the sleeves were rolled up to the middle of the forearm.

I sat in the aisle seat, exhausted. I was out of the ring and my boxing gloves lay in the briefcase under the seat. I was in the middle of reading *The Plague* by Albert Camus, a story of a French town consumed by a deadly virus. I had just read to the point where Camus describes the torturous death of a child. The doctor says to the assistant that he should contact the father to tell him of his son's death. The assistant says, "We can't. He's in isolation."

I looked up from the book into my life. Bryan had died two years earlier, but on a plane from Houston to Dallas he was dying again. I was in total isolation in a plane full of people. The weight of the day and every moment before unloaded in that moment. I never cry in public and even when I do cry I trickle more than pour. But with both book and life in hand, I wept. An uncontrollable flow of tears poured onto the page. No one noticed. The plane landed and I went home alone.

One Breath Left

When I was young the Apollo astronauts were circling the earth in preliminary flights before the lunar missions. It was the first time an astronaut had ventured out of the capsule. A white cord held him to the ship as he dangled in space. His glove came off and it floated away from him. I remember being captivated by the scene. In one of our exhausted conversations I said to Lydia, "I feel like that astronaut floating out of the ship and someone cuts the cord. I'm floating off into space, above a blue planet, away from the ship. The oxygen is gone. I have one breath left and I don't know if I should scream a soundless scream that nobody will hear or hold the breath as long as I can."

Lydia had her own metaphor. She told me, "I feel like I'm walking in a blizzard. And if I stop I die."

There were only two elements held in common in our metaphoric reflections. The first was death. The second was that we were both alone.

In that unbearable aloneness Lydia chose to move out.

In 1989, the distance in a house filled with stagnation couldn't be kept at bay any longer. Matt and I stayed in the house while Lydia rented a one-bedroom apartment three blocks away. Each day I would get Matt ready in the morning and take him to school on the way to work. Lydia would then pick him up after school and spend three hours with him until I got home. Lydia often joined us for supper. I shared the three hours before bedtime with him and put him to bed. On weekends I had Matt for Friday night rowdy and all day Saturday. Saturday night and Sunday were Lydia's turn. When I had to go out of town for business Lydia would come over to the house. We did everything we could to keep Matt's world as stable as possible.

Ironically, Lydia and I grew closer when we surrendered to the aloneness. In carving time for each other we experienced words chosen with meaning, and the depths of our conversations found a richer hue.

There were other reasons Lydia needed space, besides me, besides us. Lydia was now experiencing more specific physical deterioration. She endured pain like no other I've ever met. Of all the physical pain she experienced she said that the shingles were the worst. She calmly described it in matter of fact terms, not looking for sympathy, not even looking for understanding. How could I understand? I didn't even try. Her energy became lower and lower. She described how she felt every step was like walking in water up to her neck. There was always resistance and great effort needed just to cross a room.

Lydia didn't want Matt to see what stood before him. The times when we'd dine or go to a movie together I knew the extent of her pain and debilitation, but Matt was oblivious. Then, Lydia would reach her apartment and collapse.

She coped physically by inner emotional fortitude and mental toughness. She rose when she could and worked her job at Children's Hospital by phone when she couldn't. She would call patients who had no idea she was bedridden that day.

The Cost of a Dress

Lydia's spirit broke her before her body could. I believe it was Lydia's broken heart that took her long before her body did.

Lydia and Luke, her father, were close, as close as Matt and I were. There was a special bond between them. Both had the same reserved dignity that masked a delightfully dry sense of humor. Luke could make me laugh by the raising of an eyebrow or a casually tossed one-liner dished out with laser precision.

Luke and my father worked together for over twenty-six years. Their first job began in 1968 when my father became the pastor of First Baptist Church in San Antonio, Texas. Luke was the Minister of Education there. His quiet efficiency put the nuts and bolts together, and anything Luke put his hands to was touched with quality. As the saying goes, "the acorn doesn't fall far from the tree" and Lydia was as close to Luke as any child could be to a parent.

July 26, 1991, was Luke's sixty-fifth birthday. On July 26, 1991, Lydia's father died. A massive heart attack came out of nowhere. There were no signs, no warnings. He played tennis at least three times a week, still worked, and ate healthily.

Luke was still alive and in intensive care by the time Lydia, Matt and

I made it to San Antonio from Dallas. When she entered the intensive care to join her mother, brother and sister, Lydia didn't recognize him. The medication they gave him had an adverse effect and his body bloated. It was clear Luke had waited till Lydia, the last to arrive, was there. His family encircled his bed; each tenderly said their goodbye and Luke died on the day of his birth.

July 26, 1991, also marked the day Lydia turned towards death. There was nothing said. No pronouncements. No outpouring of a crushed spirit. But her heart broke that day. At the time, and often since, whenever I think about Luke I wonder if he left to prepare a way for Lydia.

Lydia and I went shopping for a dress. She wanted black. We left Matt with family as we went to a few shops. In her economy of energy we knew how little effort she could expend so we parked close to the mall entrance. Lydia was as unmaterialistic as anyone on the planet. We never had much money, but even if we did have some cash, which was from time to time, she still didn't do much shopping. We certainly didn't frequent the stores we were perusing the day before her father's funeral.

She lifted a dress from the rack and looked at the price. She looked at me with a half-smile. I shook my head and said, "Don't worry about the price. Do you like it?"

She laid the flowing fabric against her and looked in the mirror. "It's pretty. What do you think?"

"It's beautiful. I think you should get it."

She fingered the price tag again. "It's a lot of money."

"It doesn't matter. Try it on."

When she stepped out of the dressing room, the softness of the dress rested against Lydia's soft sorrow. Her beauty was no longer the youthful radiance that we shared the first night we laughed on her front lawn. Lydia's beauty had become weathered in wisdom. She was luminous. Her brown eyes, rimmed with dried tears, were rich and dark.

It was probably the most expensive dress Lydia had ever bought. Some moments are truly worth the price.

The dress was put in a box, not stuffed in a plastic bag. As the attendant carefully folded the dress, we both knew, but by that time words weren't needed. We knew she would only wear this dress twice — the first time to say goodbye to her father, and the second time the day after she'd say hello again.

Pandora's Box

Luke died in July. Matt and I had a trip planned in August before school started that year. Our favorite kind of trip was to jump into our little pickup and set off in no particular direction. When the day ended we'd roll our sleeping bags out on the bed of the truck underneath the camper shell. When the day began we'd roll up the bags and take the road in front of us and see where it went. We had done this through the Ozarks in Arkansas and thought it'd be a good idea to head in the direction of the Grand Canyon in Arizona.

Lydia was in no shape to be left alone. We invited her to join us on our adventure. She agreed to the terms of our freewheeling abandonment and we headed west.

It was a gift to travel with Lydia again. We headed down the same highways that took us to California in the beginning of our marriage. Here we were traveling once more, this time for the last time.

Both Lydia and I were keenly aware of the moments left. The Grand Canyon held a special place for Lydia and me. Our first anniversary was spent on the canyon's edge. We entered a magical night with a mystical sunset that colored the stone painted by sunlight. The slow sinking of the sun lifted the light up the multi-colored walls. Lydia and I held each other in the twilight of August 17, 1979. A world awaited us, the dream ready to unfold. We made love that night knowing we would wake in the morning and set off with everything we owned in the direction of tomorrow.

On August 17, 1991, we watched the eons old sunset over the same canyon. Our son sat between us, the past lay behind us, and we were running out of tomorrows. As the light danced on rocks in a repeat performance I looked over to my left. A young couple was sitting on the secluded edge of the canyon, a few feet from the road. I realized it was the same spot Lydia and I sat that August twilight in 1979.

I pointed the couple out to Lydia. A soft smile crossed her lips. I said to her, "I think I should yell to them JUMP! Don't ask any questions, just JUMP!" She chuckled a little. "Would you have jumped?"

It was my turned to smile. I shook my head softly. "No. Even if I knew all this, I wouldn't have jumped."

We stayed at the Canyon a few days. Lydia and I slept in the back of the truck and Matt was small enough to sleep in the cab. Lydia spent more time sleeping now. In the mornings, Matt and I rose first. We'd start breakfast and she would rise later. Before we started breakfast one morning, Matt and I took a stroll to see the Canyon kiss daylight. We sat on the edge looking over the majestic canyon lit in her glory. The still, cool air layered the light; we were in layers, too, in reverent silence.

I had come to a place where spirit was finding voice again. Spirit, in all her layers, began to rekindle within me again.

I knew Matt was on the threshold of his mother's death. The day would come when he would find himself in his own transition and it was time to build a vocabulary where he could speak his path. We had already begun reading Greek Mythology every night for bedtime, by his choice. He came across one book that had one god per page. It was easy to finish one a night. Matt collected many other books on the Greeks, but he always came back to that one.

My path had turned East by then. I was never to return to any organized articulation of faith, East or West, but I found a vocabulary, words that lit my path in the direction of pathlessness.

I never really understood his interest in Greek Mythology. I don't think he would have identified his path as such, but it was clear Matt had an abiding affinity to the gods that glittered in the Greek Mind.

I never tried to put my path into words for Matt either. Matt and I touched Spirit throughout our life together, an embrace here, a kiss on the cheek there. We were in Spirit at a movie or playing a video game. We watched cartoons every day, always in Spirit. And when we laughed together, we were held in the apex of Spirit. But there at the Canyon, my voice was rusty, like a hermit monk coming to a village for the first time in years. Matt's voice wasn't rusty like mine. Matt's spirit was pliable and he wore it casually in his daily movement.

I tried to keep my voice emotionally detached and ordinary, but my words were awkward as we sat on the edge of the Canyon. Matt rested against my shoulder. I said, "You know Matt, when I look out over something this beautiful, I think there must be a god out there somewhere."

I waited for Matt's reply with a tinge of trepidation. I didn't have to wait long. Matt calmly said, "Yeah, if I was a Greek I'd definitely be pissed off at Pandora."

That's all he said.

I said, "I guess you're right. I'd be pissed off at Pandora, too."

That's all I said.

One afternoon back in Dallas we were driving to his therapist. Alex had been his therapist for many years by then. Her office was right across the road from the psychiatric hospital my mother stayed in for two years when I was a teenager. I had grown quite accustomed to overlapping moments by the time of our drive.

The drive to Alex's office was nothing new; we went every week. There wasn't much to say, so we didn't. Out of our silence Matt said, "I know what the meaning of life is."

I glanced over from the road to him. He was serious. I said, "Oh yeah, what's the meaning of life?"

Matt's rich, brown eyes were soft and tired. He said, "The meaning of life is life itself."

I nodded. "That's good, Matt. The meaning of life is life itself. Where'd you hear that?"

Matt turned to the window and look out at the passing houses. "Nowhere. I just thought of it myself, just now."

Matt and I shared the meaning of life, life's true meaning in life itself. He seemed to do it naturally, by his inner nature.

The famous book, *The Tao Te Ching*, is an ancient book describing the way (Tao) and its power (Te). Some people describe the term Te as virtue, not in the sense of virtue as a moral code, but as fulfilling one's nature. Te is effortless motion. Te is the harmony of life's natural flow, flowing from the Tao.

Matt, more than anyone I've known, lived in harmony with his natural flow. It was a beautiful blend of his childlike state of innocent openness and the aged spirit that made his Te so powerful. Or maybe it was because he was dying that opened special insight into life's meaning. Or maybe it was just Matt being Matt and he didn't have the energy to be anything other than who he was. Whatever the reason, Matt was the fulfillment of his nature. The meaning of Matt's life was truly life itself.

Brothers in Arms

Matt and I shared a life and time, but Skip and I have shared a lifetime. He was two when I was born. Skip was a roly-poly kid as we called it in our childhood, soft and round with coal-black hair and hazel eyes that crinkled when he laughed. He was my forever-vigilant brother, my protector and guide. Skip was the one that held me closest. I learned, and still learn much from him.

Skip was teased and shamed a lot by other children when he was growing up. He was under siege early in life and through the years he has endured his fair share of tragedy and disaster. Many people who experience the kind of life he has walked would turn hard and cold, but Skip leans softly into moments, some quite chaotic, always carrying a gentle warmth and a sure spirit.

He can talk, joke and laugh, but he knows the value of silence as well. He never steps in uninvited. He walks tenderly when he enters a life.

My life is one of fire; Skip is as strong as water and he can curve into any moment with just the right word, or just the right silence. I'd storm the Bastille. Skip would befriend the guard, get the tour and convince the guard to let the prisoners go.

The most important thing Skip gave me during those days of hiding in our HIV was understanding. He knew what it was like to live on the outer edges of society.

Skip lived his truth, which forced him into a world of lies. I never understood why he lived so open and concealed at the same time until Lydia, Matt, Bryan and I were forced into our own underground.

Again, Skip was there to comfort and encourage. He knew what it was like to live a secret, to be an outcast. It took living in a society that spoke of quarantining my family and sending them off to some island, for me to understand what he has endured all his life.

In 1989, Skip called to tell me he'd tested HIV positive. It was my turn to sit with my big brother. I went to him and we walked the alley behind his shop. We paced more than walked. He told me of going to the Dallas County Health Department, to the same nurse that tested me. We'd get to the end of the alley and turn around to pace to the other end.

Skip didn't cry. We paced our lifetime in that alley. I don't remember the words we spoke. But underneath, layered deep, I felt the wholeness of my brother, the shared history of our travels and the tender preciousness of each moment.

Shared history was what I feared losing most if Skip died. He was the recorder of my life. Skip has a remarkable memory. He remembers conversations verbatim and minute events discarded by most. Often we would speak about our past and I'd ask if this or that really happened. If Skip, the historian, said it really happened, it happened.

He chose not to forget because he has the capacity to forgive. On many occasions Skip's water would heal my fire and I would be led to another layer by sheer love.

He told Lydia right away about his HIV. They, too, had a long shared history. They were close friends as teenagers since they were the same age and went to the same church. Lydia was one of the first people Skip told about his being gay. Lydia, in her innate equilibrium and sense of integrity, kept his secret. Now they shared something else, a common secret.

We decided not to tell Matt. Both Lydia and Matt were stable at the time. Skip was healthy as well. Matt loved his uncle deeply and we all decided to hold the illusion a little longer.

When we discussed what to tell Matt, Skip said in a matter of fact tone, "That's not a problem. I'll just tell him I got HIV just like he did, breast feeding on his mother."

Matt's boisterous sense of humor spilled over to Uncle Skip. They would tease and play, laugh and joke, hang out just hangin' out.

One night Matt and I were watching some sitcom on TV. He sat in my lap as he usually did. Two characters were gay. A gay person on TV was relatively new at that time. Matt didn't understand the joke. In explaining the joke, I introduced Matt, around eight at the time, to the world of homosexuality. I said, "The man is gay."

Matt said, "What's that?"

"That's when a man loves another man or a woman loves another woman like I love your mother."

Matt shrugged and said, "Oh."

I decided it was time. "You know, Matt, Uncle Skip's gay."

Matt never thought much about it. He never found a need to figure out why Uncle Skip was with someone named Uncle Don.

He turned his head from the TV to mine. With a crinkle in his eye and a mischievous smile, he said, "He is?"

Matt loved to tease his uncle. "Yeah, but Matt that's nothing to joke about. And you never tease someone about being gay."

Matt was disappointed. He teased Skip about everything. "Why?"

Some people have treated gay people really bad and it is cruel to joke about it."

"Why?"

"Because some people don't understand. Please, do not tease Skip."

I told Skip later that Matt knew. The next time Skip called the house Matt answered the phone. Skip said, "Hi, Matt."

Matt's voice had a lilt in the last syllable when he said, "Hello, mister gay person."

Skip broke into laughter. Matt walked the tightrope between teasing and letting his uncle know that he knew, but Matt never made jokes about Skip about being gay.

The time finally came when we decided to tell Matt about Skip's HIV status. Lydia was on the decline and we all felt we needed to tell him before her deterioration took center stage in Matt's life. It was unthinkable for Matt to discover his uncle's condition in the midst of his mother's impending death.

It wasn't as intense as telling him of his own HIV, but we did a lot of the same rounds. We prepared the family and we spoke with his therapist as well.

We decided it was between Skip and Matt. Lydia and I chose not to be there. Skip wanted to bring it up in a nonchalant manner as if it were no big deal. But it was a big deal to all of us. We had no idea how Matt would react.

Skip took off with Matt on a normal outing not unlike any other outing. Skip said that when he told Matt that he, too, had HIV, Matt nodded and thought for a moment. Then Matt said, "What time do you go to bed at night?"

A bit surprised, he answered, "About 10:30. Why?"

Matt had just started a new medicine called D4T. Matt said, "Well, you'll need to take your D4T an hour before bedtime so if you get hungry you can have something to eat before you go to sleep."
Skip thanked Matt for the advice and they went about their day as if it was just another day. In a way, I guess it was just another day for all of us.

Not Yet

I cannot imagine anything more difficult than the place where Lydia had arrived in 1991. Bryan had died five years earlier, but just minutes ago. Her closeness to Bryan encircled her with an invisible sorrow. She was moving towards death and Matt was still healthy. Standing between one child's death and one child's life, she balanced on a narrowing path. And underlying it all was the loss of her father, probably her greatest resource of strength.

Still, she continued to work at the Children's Hospital. Still, she was working to solidify the support services of the fledgling house for children with HIV. Still, she woke every day, pulled her body out of bed from a weakened spirit into a fading life.

Lydia started life with a strong spirit framed in a faith in Jesus Christ. She built her being from a genuine belief in love and service based firmly in the Christian context. Just a few days before she died we sat together in a soft night. She had long left theological conversations and theoretical beliefs behind. Her innate pragmatism had infiltrated her spirit.

She had watched children die, not just her own. Her days filled with the suffering of others in the HIV clinic and at Bryan's House.

She said to me, "I feel like evil is winning."

I asked her what she meant. She said, "Suffering is evil and evil is winning."

I said, "Lydia, I don't know any belief system in this world that believes suffering is equated with evil."

She shook her head softly, but gave no reply.

Lydia had run out of replies in the soft night's sharing, in the shadow of her death. Over a cup of hot tea I said, "I don't know if we've come to this planet to do anything. I'm clueless. But I do believe we come to learn something."

I told her what I thought I was here to learn. She nodded and said she could relate. I asked her, "What do you think you came here to learn?"

She looked into the tea that had grown cold. "I believe I've come here to learn how to let go. To let go of me. And to let go of Matt."

"And have you learned it?"

A gentle smile leaned against her weariness. She said, "Not yet."

One lamp lit the living room. We didn't have drapes and the street light left subdued streaks on the hallway. I asked her, "What do you think is on the other side?"

Her voice was soft but strong. Her eyes moved from the tea and into mine. She said, "I don't know. All I know is I'll know my babies."

"Don't Let Him Forget Me."

I called home from Washington D.C. on a November night. For the past three years I had been one of the commissioners appointed to the National Commission on AIDS (NCA). The NCA was a committee appointed to advise the President and Congress on the HIV epidemic. It began in 1988 and concluded in 1992. We were sent all over the U.S. to hold hearings so I was gone two days out of each month for four years.

Lydia always came to the house to stay with Matt when I was gone. I would call every night to speak to her and the little fella. On this night my mother answered the phone. I was surprised to put it mildly.

I asked my mother what was going on. She said, "Everything's fine. Lydia needed to go into the hospital and I'm here with Matt." Lydia was still fairly stable physically. I asked, "Which hospital?"

My mother said, "Baylor. She checked herself into the psychiatric unit." Just to hear the words psychiatric unit tumbled me into all directions. I asked, "Where's Matt?"

"Matt's right here, taking his bath. Would you like to talk to him?"

Matt was his usual chipper self. We chatted for a minute or two and he put his grandmother on the phone. I said to my mother, "I'll be home in the morning."

Lydia was not a mentally unstable person. She was one of the most balanced people I've ever known. For Lydia to check herself into a psych ward was serious. I could imagine all sorts of reasons for her seeking refuge there. Through the years she had fought the inevitable without complaint. She would tell me the latest symptom with a tone of level detachment. She was not a dramatic person to say the least. But I could imagine that under the weight of all she held inside, she had finally imploded.

There is a story of Sir Walter Raleigh weighing smoke for the Queen. The experiment entailed resting an unsmoked cigar on a scale. The cigar was smoked and the ashes carefully placed on the same scale. The difference in weight was the weight of smoke.

Lydia's life was weighed against the sorrow that had turned to ash. And the weight of the sorrow resting on the scale was becoming the only trace left of Lydia.

Psych wards are like McDonald's to me. They all look the same. The same pictures, manufactured reproductions of reproductions framed uniformly to cover white walls. Chairs, padded for protection, hospital sheets on hospital beds, TV rooms to ease the insanity and soft-soled shoes with nowhere to go shuffling hallways.

Lydia worked many years as a psych nurse. It looked foreign and surreal to see her on the other side of the glass cage. I exhaled into relief with the first look I had of Lydia. There was no trace of insanity in her. Her eyes didn't carry the look of the other side of a full moon. But her eyes were empty. She was tired, her spirit homeless.

We went to the canteen at the end of the hall. The room of soda and candy machines had four identical tables with four identical chairs. We sat there alone. She said, "I'm sorry. I just couldn't do it anymore."

Her body had turned towards death, her spirit had begun to dislodge, but she still held to the heart, her love for Matt.

She stayed in the hospital for a few more days. On a day pass we went out to a park. I said, "Why don't you come home? Do whatever you need to do to close out. And die at home."

Lydia's shoulders dropped in an audible sigh. "Oh, that would be nice. I don't want to die all alone in that apartment."

"You don't have to. Come on home."

Lydia came home to die.

She had been gone for two and a half years. Our love had space to breathe during that time. Long conversations shortened the distance. We touched memories. We drove to areas of the city that leave tracks in time and we remembered. We talked of the morrow when I would hold Matt for her; kiss him with my lips but for her spirit.

She said, "Don't let him forget me."

I couldn't even imagine the possibility of Matt forgetting her. But towards the end of her life she needed to know she did not live dreamless, alone or in vain.

We talked of how she wanted Matt to remember her. I asked her to make videotape for him. She picked *The Little Prince* and *The Giving Tree* to read to him on the tape.

We wanted to get a present for her to give to Matt. She was too tired to travel from store to store so I searched alone. In an obscure store in the West End of Dallas, a place I had never been before, there was a brass statue of three dolphins jumping out of the water. The piece was heavy and solid, strong and symbolic of the ocean that interlaced so many parts of her and Matt. I brought it home during the taping and she held the dolphins and spoke to her son of love, of remembrance.

Lydia told me that the taping of the books and the speaking of the words she left Matt were the hardest things she'd ever done. But Lydia was her usual composed self as she held the brass dolphins and spoke into the camera. No one would have known.

Final Wishes

Lydia and I met with the funeral home director in Dallas. She was a wonderful lady with a reputation of treating people respectfully. She was gentle and completely present when we spoke of Lydia's last wishes.

We met with a Unitarian minister and planned the funeral. Lydia didn't care where the funeral was held, but we wanted a ceremony for Matt. There was never a decision where Matt was not the template on which we placed our thoughts or actions. This, like Bryan's death and funeral, was more for what lay ahead for him than what was to be left behind.

Lydia was to be cremated. I asked her where she wanted her ashes spread. She said, "I don't care. It's really up to what's best for you and Matt."

I said, "How about Half Moon Bay?"

Half Moon Bay was the town just south of San Francisco. We spent many beautiful moments there. It was also where a friend had spread the ashes of his wife after over forty years of marriage.

Lydia said, "That'll be fine."

Lydia's main concern was to leave Matt with a memory, not a specific memory painted on an event, but the memory.

My memories of Lydia are of trace elements. I carry snippets, cellular snapshots that collectively become "the" memory – a laugh on the front lawn of her apartment…a rainbow we stopped to see over Point Reyes…a sunset over a canyon…ice cream…a walk in winter…walking by Matt's room as she read a book to him for bedtime…a tree we planted in the front yard in memory of a birthday Bryan never had…a memory of a memory collects into "the" memory.

I thought it was the big stuff that makes "the" memory, but the pictures pasted in my collage are of the ordinary moments: waking next to her, laughing, driving down a highway, taking Matt to the park. The "un-special" became extraordinarily special. In the last three months of Lydia's life we built a collage of moments that had settled into peace. Memory smoothed the rough edges and we sat in an extraordinary ordinariness.

In Love Into Love

I thought everything was planned. We could put it all aside and do life moment to moment. But plans changed. Lydia informed me that her mother, Joyce, wanted the funeral in a Baptist church. Joyce was not comfortable with the service being held in a Unitarian Church.

I said to Lydia, "What's her being comfortable in a Unitarian church got to do with it?"

She said, "I'm tired. I just don't want any hassles."

I leaned against the kitchen counter top with my arms folded across my chest. "So you want to have the service in a church that rejected Matt. And you don't even believe in Christ anymore."

She sat at the kitchen table. "All the more reason it doesn't matter. She's gone through enough."

"And what have I gone through?"

She looked down at the table. "I just don't have the energy to fight anymore. Please. Just let her have it. You don't like funerals anyway."

Lydia was right on all three accounts. I didn't like funerals. Joyce had gone through enough. And Lydia was too tired to fight.

Lydia's mother had just gone through the death of her husband less than a year before it was Lydia's turn to die. Joyce was close to Bryan. His death hit her hard. And not only was she to face her daughter's death, Joyce was to face the death of another grandchild.

Lydia's reserve and her way of seeing and sharing life were a reflection of Joyce's manner. When Joyce spoke she spoke her honesty in a soft voice. But much of those years she kept her silence.

Joyce's dedication to her faith was genuine and it wasn't for show that she asked Lydia to change the venue to a Baptist church. She was too real for that. Lydia said the reason was that many of the people in our background were Baptist. Luke and my father were in the Baptist ministry and it would be a place for family and friends to grieve.

Lydia's path was the path of least resistance. In her view, the spreading of the ashes that Matt and I would do was mine. The Baptist funeral was her mother's.

I believed at the time that this was the ultimate betrayal and it was a betrayal to Lydia's own genuineness of journey. Her beliefs were not in line with Christianity anymore and it was the final lie. We were still living in secret, in a lie. She was dying and no one on the outside of our small circle knew. Another lie. And now, in the time of remembrance we would be perpetuating the greatest lie of all – the disfigurement of Spirit. But I was wrong.

Just like blood rushes to the heart when physical trauma occurs, Spirit collects in the same way during loss. Non-essentials melt away. Where in a physical trauma the beat of the heart is to protect and survive, the beat of the spirit is one of opening, emptying and filling. It takes intentionality and awareness to follow its flowing pulse.

This, essentially, was our task in her last days. We took walks by the lake, watched TV, cooked dinners and did all kinds of mundane things. But all the while we were synchronizing our spirits to Spirit. In every moment a higher agenda lay dormant, ready for activation. As her body grew weaker, she saw deeper and said less. She spent her days with one of her greatest lessons as she described it – the lesson of letting go.

Deep Waters

Time afforded us time to prepare. And she used it wisely. Lydia's last months were a time of living lightly. Our days held great density and weight that only lightness could hold. We did our share of laughing and play, but that wasn't the kind of lightness that encircled us. It was the kind of lightness where water runs smooth no matter what lies under the surface.

It was a cold day in early January. Lydia and I went to White Rock Lake, to a pier next to Gaston Avenue. Leafless trees matched the barrenness of the sky. The water was dark and only the edges of the grassy bank revealed any depth beyond the surface. At the edge of the pier she stuffed her hands in the light brown overcoat and sat on the piling that rested waist high. I sat on the piling on the other side.

We had gone to White Rock Lake many times, for no reason at all, but this time the reason was Matt. Our voices were gentle, subdued.

"I'll take care of him," I said.

She nodded. "I know you will. Just don't let him suffer."

Lydia suffered. Her shingles were open and now covered most of her back and skull. She constantly coughed, spitting up mucus in tissue after tissue. Exhaustion. Dementia crept in and she was now writing everything down lest she forget. There were many more ways Lydia physically suffered, but it was on the pier that she told me about the CMV – just in passing like it was just another bit of information.

"I'm going blind. A black spot is developing in my eye."

I had known quite a few people with CMV blindness. So had Lydia. I asked, "How long have you had it?"

"A couple of weeks."

"Why didn't you tell me?"

Lydia looked at the cloudless sky, then out over the empty lake. "What's the point?"

She again said, "Take care of my boy. And don't let him forget me."

"I will. And I won't. He won't forget you…. Give Bryan a big hug for me."

She smiled. "I will."

We had more time after that day, but some days sink deeper than others and leave richer textures.

Lydia was letting go, just in time, she was letting go.

I don't know if anyone lets go in one exhalation. It seems we exhale layer after layer until the sound of breath returns to silence. She met with friends through the months, and she exhaled a little deeper. She wrote letters to the ones she would never see again, and breath found another layer's release. She wrote me a letter. "Don't open it until I die."

We exhaled another layer and a letter lay waiting.

She tried to write something to Matt, but her breath fell short. She started a journal for him and could only go three pages in before the pain became too great. Lydia's greatest challenge was to let go of Matt because she knew where he was ultimately to go. His body came from hers. And she knew he would follow her, feel the aches and pains, waste away and end in the final exhale without her. It wasn't death that Lydia could not let Matt go into; it was the torture that lay in wait for him and through which she would not be able to be there to hold him.

She had watched other children too, other tortures and other deaths at the Children's Hospital and Bryan's House. She knew what I did not.

I didn't see other children slide into dementia. I never sat with another child other than Bryan, our baby, so I was unaware of how small voices amplified the anguish. She heard the voices of children sliding into silence, into vacant stares in emaciated bodies.

It would not be her voice or the stroke of her hand over his brow during his long fevers. She would not be there to stroke Matt's back as he threw up every day.

Matt had a cough like Lydia's. After a long fit of wet, painful heaving he asked me, "Am I going to have this cough for the rest of my life?" Lydia knew she would not be there to answer him, to reassure him.

She could not say, "Matt, I will be there to hold you in what you must travel. I will kiss you at night, and when the last night comes my hand will touch your hand, my voice will rest in your ear, my breath will spread over you and we will breathe one last time together."

She knew she would have to let him go.

Returning to the Source

Matt spent Lydia's final months doing life on layers as well. On the surface he went to school, third grade. He played video games and watched TV. His physical activities were marginal, but he managed energy in spurts. He was in Cub Scouts by this age. As assistant Den Mother I was able to be with Matt. I would judge his pace and run interference when he reached a point where he couldn't keep up. He played baseball. At the age of nine, baseball was more of a battle with boredom than running after fly balls.

In deeper layers Matt watched his mother's closing down. We touched the subject rarely because there was a part of Matt that held her deterioration at arm's length. Matt liked laughter. So we laughed. Matt liked movies. So we went to movies. He liked books and making up stories so we played games around fictional characters, mythological beings swirling in worlds around mythical lands. And in the myth, under a canopy of dreams, we touched what couldn't be held, or even defined, in daylight. It was there where the hero wins; the heroine soars triumphantly into higher realms, evil dies, suffering ends and happy endings rested on pillows, under brightly colored dinosaur sheets, safe and sound in the world that wasn't the one we lived during the day.

Lydia and I had many conversations about how to prepare him, but how can anyone prepare a nine-year-old for his mother's death? He knew what death did. He knew from his experience with Bryan that he couldn't take the dirt off the grave and bring Lydia home.

For two years Matt had become reconciled to his own understanding of HIV, his own body and the increasing limitations. When she moved back home, Lydia made it a point not to hide her true condition from him. It was a time when Lydia let herself be and in the process she and Matt entered a beautiful layer of honesty.

It was incredibly difficult for Lydia to open. It was like asking a wildflower to open in the dead of winter. She was faced with her own mortality every time she faced Matt. She opened to reach deeper into Matt and, life being a composite of polarities, she had no choice but to experience Matt reaching deeper within her.

I watched a tender dance of spirits leaving signatures in invisible ink. Lydia and Matt were more involved in the business of preparing to meet again than saying goodbye. On the surface we prepared a child for the death of his mother. Beneath the surface, mother and child were two spirits preparing for another embrace. A covenant was unfolding.

She and I talked many hours of Matt's death, his final moments resting on hers. We spoke of the time we would meet again to pass son to Spirit. Lydia and I made an unspoken pact. I thought we were preparing Matt for Lydia's death. I didn't realize I was being prepared, too. By Lydia's final week everything that could be done was done. For three days Lydia entered and re-entered life. The day Lydia slipped into unconsciousness I picked Matt up from school. I said, "Mama's close to dying, Matt."

"How close?" he asked.

"It looks like soon. There's really no way to tell."

Matt looked out the windshield. I glanced over at him in his silence.

I said, "How are you doing with all this?"

He said, "Mrs. ___ (his teacher) yelled at me today. I told her I had a lot on my mind."

Matt was definitely his mother's child. I said, "Well, don't worry about that Matt. You don't need to go to school tomorrow."

He entered the house, but not her room. I said to him, "Matt, you have a choice. You can go in and see her, or you can stay here in the living room and watch TV if you want, or you can go to Grandma's. It's your call."

Matt immediately said, "I want to go to Grandma's."

My mother and father came for Matt. They each spent time by Lydia before they left with our son. Joyce and I held the vigil. There were others that streamed through the house, but by the third day we were asking for quiet and solitude.

Joyce was the only person I can imagine who could enter such a moment with solidity of spirit and healing silence. She held an unassuming space for both Lydia and me. My propensity would have been to be there alone with Lydia, but Joyce was like a drop of water that left no ripples on a still pond. She was truly remarkable.

The last time Lydia entered this world in consciousness was the last time she smiled. The hospice nurse wanted to put her on a morphine drip. Joyce asked her if she wanted the drip. I said, "If she doesn't want it, I'll take it." Lydia's last smile.

Morphine eased through the tube. A day later, the nurse said, "Her heart is still strong. It could be another couple of days." The nurse left at three in the afternoon.

I held Lydia's hand as she lay unconscious. Joyce stood on the other side of the bed. I looked at Joyce and said, "I can't make it another two days."

At three-thirty the death rattle began. Her breath started the process of emptying, transforming memory into Spirit. Joyce and I sat on each side of the bed. We knew Lydia was not going to let us go another two days. She, in death, was as compassionate as she was in life.

By this time I was sitting on the bed stroking her hair. She opened her eyes and looked into mine. Her eyes were soft, full, rich in texture. There was no fear, no holding on, no letting go. It was done. She was finished with this portion of life. Her eyes held mine and we sealed the pact in silence.

I said, "I love you." She closed her eyes. She closed her breath. And she opened into the covenant.

Joyce and I waited for the funeral director to come for the body. We took our time in the meantime, sitting in silence with her. There was a special piece of music that I played for her during her last days. I put the tape on again. Lydia liked a particular verse in the *Tao Te Ching*. Taoism wasn't her path, but she liked this one and asked me close to her death to read it to her. Again, in death, I read it by our bed in candlelight.

The passage says:
Empty your mind of all thoughts.
Let your heart be at peace.
Watch the turmoil of beings,
But contemplate their return.

Each separate being in the universe,
Returns to the common source.
Returning to the source is serenity.

If you don't realize the source,
You stumble in confusion and sorrow.
When you realize where you come from,
You naturally become tolerant,
Disinterested, amused,
Kindhearted as a grandmother,
Dignified as a king.

Immersed in the wonder of the Tao,
You can deal with whatever life brings you,
And when death comes, you are ready.

The funeral director and her husband came for Lydia's body. They lifted her off our bed. I thought back to the time of Matt's birth when I was presented with the choice of following him to the intensive care or staying with her. I walked with them to their car. They slipped her into the back and I returned to sit by our bed again. Still under candlelight with the music filling the room, I opened the letter Lydia wrote me.

Three pages, tender pages, passed.

I folded the letter and placed it back into the envelope. The music reached the end of the tape at that same moment I lay the envelope on the bedside table. I blew out the candle, rose from the chair and left to tell our son his mother was dead.

I don't know if the freeway was full or empty on the way to Fort Worth. It was dark. I remember the darkness because on the way to Matt I passed the hospital where Bryan died. The old stone building was lit from the inside, windows with other children inside.

Matt was upstairs when I entered my parents' house. He was looking at the TV, but watching me. He knew. In my eyes were her eyes, the brown eyes his mother gave him. "Matt, Mama died this afternoon."

Matt didn't respond at first. He listened, motionless on the couch. We talked for about a half an hour. He didn't cry. He didn't get hysterical or upset. He asked questions and listened.

It was time for bed. I followed Matt into the bathroom to brush his teeth. On the way, Matt said, "So Mama bit the big one."

I said, "Matt, I know this is tough on you and you don't need to push this away like that."

We slept next to each other that night in my mother and father's guestroom. I was on my back staring at the dark ceiling when I heard his muffled sniffles. I touched his cheek. He put his head on my shoulder and I stroked his hair. He finally fell asleep. I then closed my eyes, still seeing hers.

Empty Words

Another funeral loomed. The Baptist church Joyce picked was large and filled with many people wishing to pay their last respects to Lydia.

Joyce had planned the funeral with a close friend of Lydia. They had a church choir from a church that we'd never attended, in a church that never invited us, and within a belief system that no longer held meaning for us.

Eschatology is church terminology for the doctrine of last things. In my capacity as a volunteer for the AIDS Interfaith Network in Dallas I had the opportunity to listen to many eschatological ideas from people that had more than a passing fancy with the notion, unlike my years of seminary and religious studies. Just as I had asked Lydia what she thought was on the other side, I asked the people I encountered with HIV. Actually, I asked just about everybody.

I believe that a person's thoughts and actions in this plane of existence can be understood best by what he or she thinks is going to happen after death. If a person believes in a heaven and hell, then they will see, either consciously or sub-consciously, life in that context.

Fear of death is one outcome I have seen over and over in the lives of people facing "the doctrine of last things." Whenever I was with someone that faced death in fear we would venture into his or her inner landscape and they would describe their soul's journey.

They would describe the fear that was born of illusion. She or he would describe a childhood experience that shaped them, a defining moment in their "religious" understanding, a feeling that engulfed him or her in an inexplicable touch of the divine. It was like unpacking gifts brought home to family for Christmas. We unpacked a memory that may or may not have been experienced as sorrow or joy and placed it under the tree. We would play with the memory and follow its traces into the present tense. Then we would sit under the tree and I would ask, "What do you see?"

And within their words, I would see.

I didn't try to change someone's beliefs. Some thought there was a punishing God at the end waiting for them. I would share with them my belief, but gave the space for them to carry whatever they wished. In seminary I heard a definition of hell that made sense to me. My professor said, "Hell is not being separated from God. To be separated from God would mean there is something outside of God and there is nothing that can be outside of God. Hell is not separation from God. Hell is being loved by God and rejecting that love."

I sat with one soul that gripped hell too tightly. Close to death he faced what he perceived to be a vengeful God. He spoke of an unfulfilled life of failure and waste. He was losing his grip on a body, still clinging to hell. I whispered over and over, "Don't believe the lie. There is only love. Don't believe the lie. There is only love."

For a long time, however, I felt that it was God that was killing my family. It was God that took my beliefs away. It was God that took my job, my livelihood. It was God that promised love, but I did not experience it as love. My Hell, the rejection of love, was where I was. As I sat on the second row in a Baptist church for the funeral of my wife, the emptiness I felt was not love.

I tried to stay within the Christian context for many years. I worked with the CLC of the Texas Baptist and there I found authentic

Christians. I crossed paths with many beautiful Christians that reached out to us in love. I tried different denominations looking for an expression that expressed me, and I couldn't find one.

The final demise of my path in the Christian context came not so much because of how the Church treated us, but because of the way it treated those around us. Day after day I would sit with people riddled with HIV, many outside the "sanctity" of the church. They would speak of being on the outside of God, rejected. It was their rejection that finally led to my own rejection of a system that is built on exclusivity.

In seminary, many years before, I picked up a translation of Chuang Tzu's poems by Thomas Merton, a Catholic monk. I remember how it touched me then with its simplicity and clarity. The book still sat on my shelves, waiting. Spirit drew me to Spirit. This tiny collection of treasures landed under my eyes and rested in my heart. And I remembered.

It was not easy turning East. It would cost me my job. I could no longer work with Phil and the Christian Life Commission. I could have played the game of omission, but I had too much respect for Phil, and for me. This meant the loss of our insurance. And people with catastrophic illness hung in the balance of belief.

This moment of my truth came several years before Lydia died. We discussed its ramifications. She knew there is nothing more painful than the schism of a soul. She understood me and supported my resignation from the Baptist.

I went to Phil and said I needed to resign and why. Jokingly I said, "If you could change the name to Human Life Commission, I'd be happy to stay." Phil, the epitome of Christianity's best, laughed and said he wished me well. Phil loved me into my release.

When I told my father I was leaving Christianity, he cried. My words were as soft as the tears that streamed his cheeks. He could barely speak, but he knew it was inevitable. Christ isn't a word or some structural precept to him. Christ is life for him. And I was walking away from his most precious possession – life itself.

I knew what I didn't believe any longer, but until I let go of it, I would be unable to know what I would come to believe. I had to leave God to find God. There was one phrase I encountered in the leveling of a belief system that became the leaven of my expression of Spirit. It was wei wu wei. Basically, it translates as: *all action comes from non-action, stillness.* I began to be still.

Ask any refugee and they will tell you that they started the trek to freedom with more than they had when they arrived. And like a refugee, I found that the lighter I traveled the further I could go.

At Lydia's death, however, I still carried more than I could let go of for the journey. I still had old beliefs that weighed heavily on me in the pew next to my son.

The choir sang Christian hymns. Christian homilies spoke of Lydia's Christian devotion, her sacrifices to help start Bryan's House and how she eased others' pain as a nurse at Children's Hospital.

But what wasn't mentioned was that Lydia died of AIDS. She lived a painful and sorrowed life within a genuine and true spirit. She had learned to let go and she knew that love awaited her even though she no longer defined it in terms of this God or that God. This, the greatest message of her incredible life, was not shared. Lydia didn't want the HIV mentioned because she feared for Matt. The news had yet to travel through his school and she wanted more than anything for Matt to be treated normally.

I had never felt so hollow in my life. The service was not an authentic reflection of Lydia. I wanted the world to know that she won, against all, she won. She died never surrendering love. She lived giving to life. Everything had been stripped of this woman and she met her moments with dignity and grace.

I ushered Matt out of the service as soon as the last prayer ended. We walked straight down the middle aisle directly to the door and to the car. Lydia's brother, David, followed us outside. David is a good person with a good heart. If it had been anybody else I don't think I would have been able to maintain civility. He asked me if I was okay. I said, "David, I better not say anything right now." Matt and I drove out of the church parking lot back home, back to reality.

Ironically, the funeral where nothing from the pulpit was spoken about Lydia's HIV was where Matt's HIV became known. People that knew mingled with those that didn't. A word here and a whisper there ended Matt's secret. Lydia's funeral was to be the unraveling of Matt's privacy. The word was out.

A Journey of Father and Son

Matt and I left from Dallas towards Half Moon Bay, California. Lydia's ashes rested behind the cab seat of our little truck.

Lydia and I drove this road on our way to seminary. Lydia, Matt and I drove this road together. Now it was just Matt and I. One day I would drive this road alone.

Matt and I passed the Grand Canyon without stopping. I asked him if he wanted to go see it again, but he said no.

Long miles suspended me in an elongated present. Past and future sank deeper into my stillness, like a rock drifting to the bottom of a pond.

Matt and I stopped to take the tour of Hoover Dam. We swam in Lake Mead and camped at its edge. We packed up in the morning and continued on.

We played, as we always did, but as always there was, beneath the laughter, the backdrop of our task at hand. Matt and I talked about his mother, her life and her ashes. We never spoke of his ashes, but underneath the snuggles and the sorrow it shadowed us both. We talked about treatments and different medicines the scientists were working on and how they may come up with something.

Matt rode many miles in silence in the seat beside me. Just as when I matched Matt's breaths in the intensive care on his first day of life, I matched Matt's silence. When he wanted to speak, we would speak, but he had the room to roam his own thoughts, settle deep within his own journey, and wander the realms of his own spirit. I sat next to a child, next to the depths of Spirit.

I knew, even then, the futility of trying to pack more into the illusion of time. We were unpacking, not packing, memories. We drove in the direction of the sea that would hold his mother's ashes. We did not reach for what wasn't there. There was a softness that shaped us both in the days spent on the road. We approached San Francisco at night. Light glittered the distinctive skyline. Matt was asleep as we passed the city and moved towards Pacifica. I was not prepared for the moment at hand. I did not seek the experience; but like other experiences I was drawn to its center.

Matt and I entered the tunnel with intermittent lights, the one where I looked over at Lydia in seizure with her eyes rolled back, blood dripping down the side of her mouth, her hands flailing against the dash and her face appearing and disappearing between light and dark. I touched Matt's leg as his face shone in the light and was lost to the darkness.

I looked into the present dream sitting asleep beside me. His breath was gentle and steady. Traces of peace illuminated in light and rested in dark.

Lydia's ash silhouetted us. I did not see my son in that tunnel. I saw our son, our child that I was to raise, to teach in the ways of life, and to guide into the ways of death. Our son slept beside me, in our dream. And in the millisecond between light and dark Lydia and I met in the tunnel to caress our son, her in our eternality, and I in our brevity.

X Marks the Spot

Half Moon Bay stretches a long sandy beach across her edge. A small harbor leans against the north end. Sailboats, fishing boats and other vessels rocked softly against the wooden pier when Matt and I went to meet the man that was to take us out to sea. The old hippie was a friend of a friend. He had long, thinning gray hair. His weathered face was gentle. He lived on his sailboat so we entered his home. He entered our task with sacredness.

The sun was unobstructed. The sea was calm and windless as we puttered by motor out of the harbor. A mile out to sea we stopped. I opened the cardboard box and pulled out the thick plastic bag. Matt studied the ash. I had asked him before if he wanted to see it and he said no. This was his first sight of what was left of his mother's body. I watched him study the sealed bag.

Matt finally reached in and held his mother's ash, but he watched me and my reactions. His breath was synchronized to mine and he was keenly aware of the need to see just how I treated death.

The captain was quiet and slid into the background. Matt and I leaned over the side of the boat that faced the shore. We took turns in wedding ash to sea. His small plump hand dipped into the bag and he lifted it into the air as if to delay its fall into the cold waters of the Pacific. I poured my portion of her as close to the sea as I could as if to lay her softly in her bed.

We didn't know what to do with the bag. A film of ash that clung to its edges left us both uncomfortable. Matt and I decided we would dip the bag into the ocean. We both held the bag as we poured the ashen sea back into herself.

It was up to us as to when to return to shore. The man at the helm made no move until we asked. He started the engine and we puttered slowly back to harbor. He took his time, reverently so. Matt and I lay down in the front of the boat, his head resting on my chest.

The captain docked his home at the pier. Before we left he handed me a weathered nautical map of the bay. The edges were frayed and stained yellow where it had been folded. It was all he could give us beyond his gift of silence. He made a small x in pencil where Lydia's ash disappeared. I folded the map, shook his hand and walked Matt to the car.

Matt and I sat for a while looking out over the ocean at Half Moon Bay. We didn't stay for sunset. We'd already seen it.

Monterey – Going Once, Going Twice

The next day Matt and I headed for a day trip down to Monterey. Lydia, Matt and I had been there several years earlier. The most beautiful aquarium sits between the city and the sea. In fact, part of the aquarium is in the sea. We had created a lovely memory on that trip in 1987.

Monterey was a memory of another time as well. Lydia and I had spent our honeymoon in San Francisco in 1978. We did all the romantic touristy things newlyweds do. One collection of memories was our journey to Monterey. The aquarium had not been built then. The memory that I kept was of the indoor merry-go-round in the tourist area of Monterey. It was a fun evening empty of all that awaited us. She sat on the brightly colored merry-go-round. When she laughed, she sparkled.

When Matt and I drove past Half Moon Bay on our way to Monterey he looked out the window. I waited for him to speak. He didn't. We entered the aquarium for a second time, but for the first time without Lydia. Sharks swam close to the edge of the thick glass. Sea lions swirled in a graceful dance, eyes wide open, revealing an ancient vastness. Outside, we sat theater in the round style to watch the feeding of otters and sea lions that came from the open sea into the show. We did everything we had done before, but for the first time without Lydia.

I put Matt on the brightly colored merry-go-round. And when he laughed, he sparkled.

Small Ripples in a Large Ocean

Lakewood Elementary students ranged from the wealthy to the poor. Matt sat in the middle. Since Lydia's funeral, news of Matt's condition began filtering out. It wasn't like wildfire, but there was a growing suspicion and a few whispers here and there.

Matt and I talked about whether to go public or not. We went over the pros and cons of letting the world in on his secret. I knew it was a matter of time, as most matters are. Matt's health was still stable and he looked good despite his steady decline.

He was well-accepted in school during this period of secrecy. Other students treated him as one of their own. His laughter and wicked sense of humor kept him in good stead with the mischievous ones and his innocent good-natured spirit attracted other good-natured kids. Lydia and I had worked hard to get the system to know and accept Matt, but Matt was Matt's greatest asset.

I felt it was time to share our situation for several reasons. The first reason was that Lydia and I had agreed that when the school at large caught on, we would take the offensive and present our case in the view of public opinion. We felt that if the spotlight was on Dallas, Dallas had a better incentive to behave favorably to Matt.

The second reason was I did not want him to have to live in secret. Matt's emotional and physical health would be enhanced if he could just be normal in the midst of our abnormality. He was going to need his energy to live with the increasing illness and he didn't need to spend his days hiding his condition.

The third reason centered on what we could give back. I had been traveling the country with the National Commission on AIDS (NCA). We did hearings and site visits in large cities and small rural communities. It was not difficult to identify with all of the spectrums of HIV's devastation, but the one that weighed in strongest in why I felt it was best to "come out" was rural Georgia.

South of Macon, Georgia, is peanut country. Agriculture spans the land and small towns lie scattered between lines of fields and forest. The HIV epidemic's tentacles reached deep into the sociological, psychological as well as the physical dimensions of life. We heard stories of rejection and fear, isolation and secrecy, not unlike their counterparts in metropolitan areas. But it was the isolation and distance of the Deep South that hit me most. We heard voices of poor families hiding adult sons in back bedrooms, mothers hiding with their small children, terrified of other parents and school systems. People with no power whispered their tales to me.

My family was not unique, but we were in the unique position to speak.

Matt and I spoke of the cons. We didn't know what kind of reaction he would receive. I talked to Matt about how people like Ryan White had paved the way for people like us. I told him what Lydia said many years ago – "Someday people will catch up with facts." Matt liked that.

He said he was ready. I spoke with the publicity person at the NAC. He set up a phone interview with a reporter from the *New York Times*.

I don't remember the reporter's name, but I remember the feel of his voice. It was steady and unassuming. He felt to be a good man. I told him our story and he asked a lot of questions. He listened and in the process he found the angle. It wasn't sensationalized and he did a good job at simply reporting the facts, but I was disappointed in the focus of the article.

I wanted the article to be more on what we had done to give back to life in the midst of our tragedies. I wanted the article to center on Lydia's work with Bryan's House and Children's Hospital. Lydia had served on the first Congressional funding for Dallas. She had dedicated many hours to the needs of others. The reporter also could have written about how I had participated with the AIDS Interfaith Network, the Texas Legislative Task Force on AIDS, and now the National Commission on AIDS. By that time I was working for pay with the University of Texas Southwestern Medical School in the HIV Research Department. I worked as a liaison with Parkland Hospital, the school and the community, and he could have written about the care still needed for people like us.

I wanted him to write about Matt. How a nine-year-old lived life to the fullest within the slimmest of circumstances. I wanted those in places like rural Georgia to not feel so alone. I wanted other schools to accept their children that lived in hiding, families that held something worse than the disease – the silence of disease.

I wanted the reporter to share about all the good people we encountered along the way. How just as many people of spirit rose to meet us with compassion and love as those that rejected us. Even though the churches had turned their back, there were plenty of Christians who helped us.

But the reporter chose another angle. It was the truth, but not the truth I wanted.

The *New York Times* wrote of the treatment we received from the church in Colorado when we first found out. He wrote about the churches in Texas that turned us away.

I opened the *Times* that morning to the front page and read the article like anyone else would. My heart sank, but at least the secret was over. We had prepared the school. The principal had a statement. The teachers were ready. Matt was ready. I just wasn't ready for the response.

Parents called in support. Classmates rallied around Matt. When the secretary told us three years earlier that we would "regret the day we enrolled Matt into Lakewood Elementary," she was wrong. Open arms encircled Matt.

There was one parent that participated in everything and was at the school quite often. She carried confidence and a powerful presence. She was energy personified and when she walked in the room I would secretly tremble. For years I cowered in the thought of what would happen if she found out. She had a radiant smile, but I had no desire to be on the other end of a frown from her. She was one of the first to call. My fears were unfounded. Her natural propensity to organize and coordinate turned to us, big time. To the end of Matt's life she was one of the ones that carpooled kids to the house to see him. Her heart equaled her energy. If there were to be any opposition to Matt being in that school they would have had to face a calm and extremely competent principal, loving teachers, many supportive parents, and Vicki. As far as Matt was concerned, God help the one that crossed Vicki.

Matt and I held an information session for parents and classmates. Janet came to give the medical facts. Matt shared Matt. The students listened, asked questions. Matt and his gentle spirit were his answers.

Surfing a Tsunami

I was not ready for what ensued beyond that initial public revelation. Once the *New York Times* set the wheels in the motion describing how the church treated one of its own, there was no way to derail that train. Breaking news is like a tsunami. I felt like a tidal wave had hit and all we had was a surfboard.

We were inundated with TV news and newspaper reporters. And we just had to ride the wave till it ran its course. The news world is an interesting phenomenon – it's a house of cards playing each card as quick as it can.

Belinda had warned me. Belinda Mason was one of the initial commissioners on the NAC. The Congressional legislation originating the Commission dictated that a person living with HIV must be appointed. Belinda was that person. Her natural red hair was as thick as the Kentucky drawl that hid her quick mind and quicker sense of humor. One of Belinda's finest qualities was "what you see is what you get." She was a fast read of any situation, clear and concise. She would tell you what she thought in simple language, and her simplicity revealed deep truth and wisdom.

I watched Belinda being mobbed by the press looking for a story to fill the nightly airwaves. They would pounce on her and in a slow drawl she drew them a picture with eloquent words – sound bites to them, heart to her. We sat in her hotel room after one of the onslaughts of the tsunami. I was terrified of this pack of cameras and pencils. In a matter of fact tone and a wry smile, she said, "It's like being f---ed without being kissed."

The first time I really got to know Belinda was early in the Commission's work. We were both speaking at an HIV conference in Sante Fe, New Mexico. She walked with great discomfort. The infection was not kind, gentle or slow for her.

If anyone could tell me what it was like for Lydia, it would be Belinda. She had two children and a husband that weren't infected. She was about the business of losing her family, just like Lydia. She was doing her best to give back to life, just like Lydia. We talked into the night. I listened to a wise woman who told it the way it was. We talked more about the press and what it took as opposed to what it gave.

Her exhaustion showed. She said, "Sometimes I feel if I told them what it is really like I'd just start screaming and not be able to stop." Yet, I watched Belinda touch lives, not just those living with HIV. She treated every reporter, every person, as if they were special, which can only come from a special person, as it is impossible for that to be artificially manufactured.

There are two sounds that still echo – Lydia's death rattle and the sound of the Kentucky clay that ricocheted off Belinda's casket.

Belinda and I had the same flight from New Mexico back to Dallas. I was exiting in Dallas and she would head on to Kentucky. We were not assigned adjoining seats. I asked the man in the aisle next to Belinda if he would change seats with me. I had an aisle seat, too, and I thought it would be no problem. The portly man in the uniform of business said, "No, I'm happy where I am."

I know the value of time and time lost. The man underscored the cost of complacency. A whole presidency went by before HIV was even mentioned by a Commander in Chief of the United States. Belinda and

I were there when President Bush finally gave the first speech on HIV in March of 1990. She spoke that day – pure Belinda. It was to a crowd of business people. I sat in the audience thinking of the man on the plane and all the words of a very wise woman I missed that day.

The press moved quickly. Matt and I ended up in New York and on TV's *The Today Show* – ushered in, ushered out. We met with Jane Pauley and agreed to be interviewed. I had no idea how invasive it would be until our house was teaming with cameras, lighting, wires and people. The poor producer of the show had to contend with my perpetual reluctance. Jane was tender and kind. She was not like the ones I saw take a bite out of Belinda and head off to lunch on the next headliner. Jane entered our world with respect and left with respect.

Others reporters came and went. And each time I thought about where we were when I first heard Ryan White and what it meant to me. I'd think of rural Georgia. And I hoped that somewhere someone wasn't feeling so alone.

Matt was safe. The school went beyond any expectation I ever could have imagined. The handful of parents who distanced their children from Matt paled in comparison to the many that embraced him.

Most importantly, he was able to be real. When he was sick he could rest without excuse. As the days lessened the years, as his spirit grew and his body declined, the children he grew up with at Lakewood Elementary grew with him. Matt sat in a classroom of kids no longer alone.

Just Out of Reach

There is a difference between being alone and loneliness. I had known Lydia since I was eleven. We were married for fourteen years, parented two children, drifted in and out of love and came to a place love could only dream of. Now I was alone, and the loneliness of the years she lived a few blocks away converged with the aloneness.

A month after Lydia's death I met someone. I had an expectation that after all I had been through that I would find someone who I would spend the rest of my life with, and they would know Matt and we would grieve together when he died. As if I would be rewarded for going through hell by having a taste of heaven.

The relationship lasted a year and a half, including a six-month marriage. What I thought I could do, I could not. I could not walk into a new life carrying the old one so close. It was an impossible task for both of us.

What I found typified in that experience was that no matter how much I wanted to move on I was unable to find the way out of what I was in. I tried other relationships and I carried into them the same shadows. I was unable to place love for another over what Lydia and I experienced. No matter how much I yearned for something to be different, for me to be different, I was who I was and it was impossible to be anything other than who I was in relationships. It is like the phrase *wherever you go, there you are*. Also, I found in my economy of energy that there was only so much I was able to do. This was the case in relationships, in work and all points in between.

While I was working at the medical school I read a study about the productivity level for caregivers and families of terminal patients. I don't remember the statistical data, but I remember the relief I felt when the study articulated the diminished productivity of the caregivers in their jobs. I always felt I was barely able to do the basics. I thought making it to the office was a minor triumph. I knew I could do more, but I couldn't. It's like someone who played superior tennis as a young man, lets the game go and then tries in middle age to play again, all the while wondering why he can't play like he used to. Life was a struggle between what I thought I *should* be able to do and depleting resources to do it.

The two-day monthly travels with the Commission, the barrage of press, my job and various speaking engagements weighed heavy. I yearned for equilibrium. My life had worn thin. Everything seemed just out of reach.

Shoes, Holy Ground
and Washington, D.C.

Washington D.C. is the largest amusement park in the world. It's quite a ride. The price of admission was for me too great. There are players and there are spectators. I was one of the spectators. I met people of power – the President, the Speaker of the House, the Senate Majority Leader, other senators and representatives, great scientists and other very, very "important" people. None of whom would remember me. The two-day excursions of the NAC took us to Washington when we weren't visiting sites around the country. There are three memories I treasure the most from my four years of trips to Washington – a dinner with my father, a visit to the Holocaust Museum with Matt, and a blossom from a cherry blossom tree.

My father had business in Washington during one of my trips there. We didn't get to spend a lot of one on one time together during those years. When I was a child my father would take each of us three children on one of his business trips once a year.

I still give him grief about one particular year when he took Skip to Los Angeles and visited Disneyland, Mike went to Washington and took a tour of the Capitol, and I got to go to Dalhart, Texas, and ride a Pullman train back to Dallas.

We were going off to Williamsburg, Virginia, for a couple of days of alone time. It was a welcome reprieve. I was tired in emotion and body. The dinner was special, but it wasn't the dinner that kindled the moment of memory. Our conversation drifted to a variety of topics. Our words, as they usually did, drifted to Matt. Tears began to well up in his eyes. He said, "You are the best father I've ever seen."

I have failed in a lot of areas in my life, but if there is one thing I know, it is that with all my failings, I was a good papa. I stood bridged between two generations in that dinner. The repercussions of his kind words spread over me. My father's love for his son was the same love I had for my son. Some surreal moments are as real as they come. I glimpsed the world through Matt's eyes as I was reminded what a father means to a son. It was like finding two pieces of a massive puzzle fitting together.

The second treasured memory was experiencing the Holocaust Museum with Matt. I had been there once before with the NAC so I was prepared for what Matt would see, and I wanted Matt to see it. Matt was eleven in age and centuries old in wisdom.

We talked quite a bit about going. I told him of the tragedy that took place in the war and what was in the museum. He thought about it and said he would like to go.

I watched Matt's movement – the movement of his eyes, the movement of his mind, the movement of his heart. He whispered to me, "Why would people do this to other people?"

There was a walkway over a sea of shoes, shoes taken from the people as they were sent to be gassed. Hundreds and hundreds of shoes. Lives filled those shoes. I stood on the walkway with my arm around Matt. A bush that burned rose in my mind. God said to Moses, "Take off your shoes, you're on holy ground." Shoeless, these people stepped into sacredness, moved into the One, the holiest ground of all.

I thought of the day after Bryan was buried and Matt, three years wise, began taking clumps of dirt off his little brother's grave. The memory returned of when I explained why we couldn't take Bryan home – that when we swim we take off our shoes because we no longer need them.

The journey of shoeless souls under a walkway of Spirit gave testimony.

Matt walked out of the Holocaust museum deep in thought, still settling into the expanse of what he just encountered. It was an important moment. I wanted him to know that we carry a common path with common dangers, that the world carries darkness as well as light, and each and every human carries the world.

My last treasure in all those years going to Washington was a blossom on a cherry blossom tree. The tree sat within a row of trees in a concrete city. There was nothing out of the ordinary about this tree. From a distance it looked like all the other trees in the symmetrical orchard, but up close it was unique. The shades of bark were hers alone. The blossoms curled and swayed in the caressing breeze as no other could. Her limbs stretched both out and up like a dancer's shining encore.

This particular blossom blended with the other blossoms. It was the sunlight, the breeze and the way she fluttered that drew me into her. This cherry blossom reminded me of what I never wanted to forget.

Washington doesn't dine, it devours. And every time I entered the halls of power I felt its insatiable hunger. This anonymous blossom stood in contrast to concrete, in testament to both softness and seasons.

I felt particularly devoured that springtime day. The Commission had just endured another round of statistical data, voices proclaiming they weren't statistics, policies and procedures, power and powerlessness. In some moments it washed over me. But on occasion the words twisted like a spear lodged between the heart and lung.

There was something about the resilient fragility of the way the wind lifted the blossom. I sank into her after the long day. The deeper I went, the more I trailed her plight, and the further I went from microcosms to macrocosms. The blossom hung on a limb that grew from a trunk, rooted in earth, spinning on an axis of a round ball that moved around a sun, which, in turn, moved in an orchard of galaxies. It was a simple and profound reminder.

There was a time when I thought of my future. The job at the medical school was never going to be permanent. I could have parlayed some type of employment in the world upon whose edge I danced in Washington. It was a blossom on a cherry blossom tree that reminded me of me and how I was to travel a different path.

To Go the Distance

The more complicated life gets, the simpler I take it. The crazier it got on the outside the more I rested on the inside. Given the choice between shaping public policy and watching cartoons with Matt, I'd take the latter in a heartbeat.

Where Matt went I was to follow. It was my only desire to clothe his spirit as he shed his skin. I thought I could do relationships. I thought I could do a better job at work. I thought I could juggle and balance the exterior world. But I could not. Something had to give.

I made a conscious decision not to shut down, not to protect any part of me from him. I thought I was well-versed in what that entailed, but in reality I had never actually crossed that line where there is nothing to hold on to, nothing held back; where there is only love.

I chose to walk completely next to Matt's spirit, with freedom in his freedom. My only desire was to go the distance, to be fully present in each moment until the moment when, for Matt, I would end and Lydia would begin.

For a long time, I would wake up each morning in utter dread. I would look at Matt and all I could see was that he was going to die. I kept seeing his funeral and the day after our last day. But slowly, I began the alignment of spirit in the journey of stillness. I began waking up each morning and saying to myself, "Yes, he's going to die, but not today." Then we would live that day, only that day, to its fullest.

My journey moved in another direction. Perhaps I could have raised a notch on the employment food chain in the Washington milieu, but I had a more important task. My job was to watch cartoons, go to movies and hamburger joints, and read books to Matt at nighttime.

My real job description was to open, to follow the interior lining of life and do whatever I could not to close down or shut out anything. If I closed, Matt would have closed. If I spent a day in fear of the day after the day he died, so would Matt.

I was teaching Matt how to die. Matt was teaching me how to live.

The Eye of the Hurricane

"Where Does the Sky Begin?" was the title of a sermon by a Unitarian minister in the mid-1800s. I have chewed on the title for over twenty-five years.

Where does the sky begin? Is it just centimeters, or millimeters above a blade of grass? Is sky defined by what isn't sky? What is sky?

Where does loss begin? Is it just centimeters or millimeters from where the heart meets breath? Is loss defined by what isn't loss? What is loss?

Did my loss begin with the phone call from the blood bank in 1985 or some moment long before? I don't know. My loss lives in relation. It has to have other to be loss. The difficulty has not been loss, but discerning its distinguishable marks with precision and clarity.

Lydia came in the bedroom one night after Bryan died. She caught me in tears. I said to her, "I don't know if I'm crying for Bryan, or for you, or for Matt or for me."

Preparatory loss is a different texture than grief painted by a past loss. Losing felt more ethereal than the tangibility of loss.

But the grief process confused me, kept me off balance as it pressed against my daily life. I had a tremendous difficulty in discerning what I felt, the origin of the feeling, beginnings and endings of a thought, a feeling, and a moment.

The metaphor that describes my life during my initial years of intense loss was that I felt like I was hanging onto a tree in a hurricane. The bark of the tree tore my skin, but I couldn't let go. The gale force winds hurled heavy objects into me, but I couldn't let go. I held tighter as each thought, each event, each moment perpetually bashed me between the hurricane and the tree. Every day I just hung on for dear life.

Then the eye of the hurricane passed over me. And there was my moment of truth. I could either let go of the tree and follow the stillness of the eye, or hold on as the stillness moved on and the torrential winds tore at me again. It would appear on the surface to be a no-brainer, but hurricanes were what I knew best. Stillness was a foreign commodity to me.

I began the journey of stillness in 1989. I made the choice to let go of the tree and follow the eye of the hurricane wherever it led. I let go of fighting what isn't and settled into what is. I gave up trying to fit into a spiritual system that didn't work for me. I let go of alcohol because it inflamed the fire rather than cooling the turbulent waters. I let go of an occupation that did not reflect the path. I examined my life and found the only way to make the outside work was to release into the inward journey through stillness and effortless motion. And when I started aligning my inside with what is, my exterior began reflecting the harmonic balance between stillness and motion.

Stillness teaches me effortless motion and effortless motion teaches me stillness.

Layers of the Shell

After his mother died, Matt's stillness took the form of night. It was a restless stillness. We read our nightly book of Greek mythology, turned on the sound of humpback whales, turned out the light and I would leave. This was when Matt cried, when he had run out of thoughts and he was left with the underlying current of loss. I waited for a moment or two outside his door. Matt's sniffles turned to wails. I opened the door, climbed to the top of his bunk bed and descended next to him. His cheeks were drenched and his eyes stayed fixed on the ceiling. Pressed against one elbow I lay on my side by his side and stroked his hair. Occasionally he glanced over at me and then his eyes again locked magnetically against the white wall above us.

When Matt's gaze moved back into the room, back to the bed and into my eyes I asked, "Do you want to talk about it?"

Where does the sky begin? Was Matt crying for his mother, for Bryan, for me, or for himself? What part of his sorrow did I step into? I would have been a fool to guess. Matt wailed, "I miss Mama."

We collected memories like seashells on sand. We stroked each memory with tenderness like a child's hand on the edge of the detailed layers of the shell. Then Matt would fall asleep.

In his sleep I slowly lifted myself off the squeaky bed and descended the wooden ladder. In the dark I walked through a minefield of toys and books to the hall light that squeezed under the door. I always took one last look at Matt while the light poured into his dark room. I stood in the doorway to listen to his breath and make sure he was asleep; matching breath for breath, I closed the door.

Who Will Stop for Matt?

One of Matt's sixth grade school assignments was a handout with the question, "What are three major accomplishments you would like to achieve?" Matt wrote: 1) graduate from elementary school, 2) graduate from junior high school, and 3) graduate from high school.

In an education system where those who don't keep up get left behind, we experienced something unique at Lakewood Elementary. Matt slowly and steadily fell behind physically and mentally. Dementia inched its way into Matt, stealing small portions of his mind at first, increasing as death approached. Medically, dementia closes the mind's capacity to remember, to retain. It is amnesia by attrition, a daily decline into the forgotten, but its cruelty is that the mind knows that the mind can't remember. By sixth grade, Matt's mind weaved between two worlds and it was painful to watch his sharp mind slip into its inevitable erosion.

It was Lydia's greatest fear for Matt. At the end of her life she had to write everything down, have a timer to remember to take her medication and cover the forgotten as best she could.

One memory of Lydia stands at the forefront. Matt was eight, a year away from her death. We had all of Matt's cognitive skills tested in an extensive process to determine if the HIV was affecting his mental capacity. The researchers wanted to see the extent of what the virus did on a brain. We wanted to see the level of our child's capability so we could determine the level of parenting we needed to give Matt to ensure his most optimal experiences, including school. If he was unable to do a certain level, pushing him was the last thing we wanted.

Lydia and I listened to the researchers describe Matt's condition. At the age of eight, Matt still had a normal range of mental abilities and cognitive skills. We were both relieved, but Lydia more so because she knew what I didn't.

Life had worn Lydia threadbare. But when we got in the car she was exuberant. Her gestures were crisp and not weighted with conscious effort. Her voice lifted with a resonance of delight I had long forgotten she once possessed. Her lightness broke the shadowy weariness that clouded her and she glittered with a shining brightness. It was as if Lydia was Lydia again.

Her child was normal. It wasn't just that he was able to function on a third grade level. It was more. His path wasn't hers, yet.

But at the age of twelve, Matt's path was now hers. School was now a place to be among his friends. On his better days he attended class, but the nights of homework were long gone.

There were two steps to the front porch and door at our home. At first Matt could take those two steps with ease. I measured the moments left by those steps. A time came when he would steady himself on my arm. Then, I would hold him and we would take one step at a time. I remember the first time I carried him over the two steps. His wheelchair rolled easily, bouncing slightly from the lower step to the second and onto the porch. I measured our moments by those steps.

I remember watching one of the Special Olympics races on TV – the children's sprint. Mentally challenged children burst out of the starting blocks with focused determination. Sadly, one of the runners fell. But instead of running on past him, the other competitors stopped to help the fallen one to his feet. It moved me deeply to see such compassion. It was the greatest testament of what human beings are actually capable of being.

Who will stop for Matt?

Physically, Matt was depending more and more on the wheelchair. The other kids were growing up while Matt was growing in. But Lakewood Elementary, from the principal, teachers, parents and students, did not leave Matt behind. Matt's six years at Lakewood were another great testament of the best humanity has to offer. It lends hope to what is possible.

They did a lot for Matt; some quite spectacular events were organized. Lakewood started an award for the most distinguished student in the sixth grade class called the Matt Allen Award. Matt was its first recipient.

They put together a day called the Circle of Life. Every school grade from first to sixth surrounded Matt with flags, entering the black top in the back of the school to Elton John's song, *The Circle of Life*. Teachers and friends of Matt spoke about what Matt meant to them. Matt rose from his wheelchair and held on to me as he slowly ascended the steps to the microphone. His speech was unprepared; he spoke his heart. He said, "Students and teachers, thank you for all the support you've given me and my family. It has meant so much to me and them. And please do the same for any other child that may be HIV positive that comes to this school."

A tree was planted and dedicated to Matt in the front of the school. The same school that terrified me in our silence every time I let him off in the morning was the same school that stopped for Matt and didn't leave him behind.

Moon Over a Still Pond

I believe a society is defined by how it treats the ones it is easiest to leave behind. How we treat the aged, the ill, the poor, the fallen is the mark of who we really are. Growing up within the lens of Spirit taught me that it is not what I have that gives meaning. I was taught what I did with what I had was the measure of meaning.

Matt had an unconscious ability to draw others into a place of meaning. He just did life, played video games, watched TV, went to school and hung out. He didn't try to be something he wasn't. Matt seemed to settle into what he was and his authenticity was infectious. Yet, there was more.

Walk into any hospital ward housing terminally ill children and it is like walking into a golden light, an unearthed hidden treasure. There is something about a child's capacity for sacred simplicity. Ancient wisdom seems to settle on the souls of such creatures.

Every month for almost ten years, Matt went for treatments of gamma globulin. It was a two-hour process with an intravenous feed. Children's Hospital in Dallas had a wonderful staff. We would see other children from time to time. What emanated from these children woke me to what emanated from Matt. It wasn't what was said, or even done, by the ones standing in the light of death. It was the ordinary way these children carried the extraordinary. It wasn't an innocence Matt carried that humbled me. It was his capacity to lean into the layers with an innate knowingness.

Matt was the epitome of the moon's reflection over a still pond. It was his stillness that reflected in the busyness of a world that buzzed around him. It was in this interchange with Matt that people saw themselves, the better of themselves. It was fascinating to watch people enter Matt's life. Each person, whether consciously or unconsciously, touched a deeper part of themselves in the process.

Death is but a window. And through a child the window is clearer.

I was conscious of Matt's power within me the first time I rubbed Lydia's womb and Matt moved. I was aware of my reflection as his finger wrapped around my hand in the intensive care his first night on this side of that. I was keenly aware of where Matt touched me and the infinite extent of that touch. But in the last years of Matt's life, his sixth year at Lakewood Elementary, I watched others touch and be touched by this child. And I realized that it wasn't just because I was his father. It wasn't even because it was Matt. It was because meaning, true meaning touched the transcendent with transcendence in us all.

Autumn and Falling Leaves

I don't know when the moment unfolded. When does a leaf know when it is time to let go?

Morning before dawn was my time to ready the day.

The candle was soft, the air still. In the room spirit collected into Spirit. There was presence circling the morning stillness. I wanted to speak to Lydia again. I wanted to know. How did she do it?

The candle's dance of light lifted where she once sat. Flame flickered into light and then retreated to darkness like a wave that rolls to shore, touches sand and slides back into herself again. How did you do it, Lydia? How did you let go of Matt?

The University of Texas Southwestern Medical School gave me a leave of absence with pay and medical insurance for the last year of Matt's life. Outside of a cure, there was no greater gift I could have been given.

Donna was Matt's hospice nurse. She was very experienced in working with children. She thought he had only a few months to live when she first started. She came every week for over nine months.

Letting go takes what it takes. The fact that Matt lived longer than anyone's expectations was not a tribute to his fortitude or my care.

In retrospect, it was more of an indictment to my inability to let go.

A reporter asked me in a tactful way as to why I thought I didn't get infected and they did. In other words, why I lived and they died. I said to him that I didn't see me staying alive as the one who won. We journey till the journey is finished. They were able to finish earlier than I was.

I was not finished. Candlelight reflected my curse of wanting one more day, one more night, one more moment.

Donna was mystified by the way Matt and I spent our days. I would pack Matt up every morning and head for a fast food restaurant for breakfast, pull out the wheelchair and wheel him in. He could only take two or three bites of a hash brown. I read him the scores and standings of his beloved Atlanta Braves. We'd pack up and I'd drive slowly back to the house by way of White Rock Lake.

Matt and I had no intention of waiting for death. We were going to do what we could while we could. Death knew where to find us. We didn't see any need to hang around for it.

"I've Loved You All My Life."

Matt wanted to live to be a teenager. On October 4, 1995, he turned thirteen. Vicki rounded up some of Matt's classmates. Barbara and Kurt brought Alison and Zack, Matt's best friend to the party. And there was Kate.

Matt fell in love with Kate when he was around six, but had never told her of his love. I did not know Kate or her parents. They traveled in different circles. I called Kate's mother and told her the situation. I asked her if she wouldn't mind bringing Kate over if Matt wanted to see her. I had yet to ask Matt just in case Kate's parents didn't want her to come. She said she would talk it over with Kate and get back to me. She called back shortly and said they would love to come over.

Kate and her mother entered the living room. Kate was a beautiful young girl. Matt had good taste. She had long brown hair, lovely features that became even lovelier when her shyness gave way to a smile.

She didn't know Matt was so in love with her. It was an awkward moment I would just as soon have missed. Matt was emaciated and the dementia came and went. I had no idea what condition he would be in at this point. We were in the midst of sharing pleasantries when Matt blurted out, "Kate, I've loved you all my life."

Kate was gracious. She did not feel the same, but she said, "Thank you, Matt."

Matt said, "Can I kiss you on the cheek?"

I was crawling out of my skin. Kate's mother smiled when Kate looked over at her. Then Kate leaned close to Matt and he kissed her on the cheek.

My relief was short-lived. Matt said, "Can I kiss you on the mouth?"

Kate eyes jerked towards her mother. I jumped in and said, "I think that's enough for now."

Kate was relieved. Her mother was cool and tenderly understanding. We talked for a while longer. Matt became tired and he went back to bed.

As I was helping Matt into bed I said, "Well, how was it?"

Matt said, "It was great."

Matt was glad to see Kate made it to the party.

The first time I saw the extent of Matt's emaciation was at his birthday. I had already been battling his bedsores that were caused by the lack of muscle between skin and bone. I dressed them every day and rotated him through the night. Yet, I still didn't see his body's demise.

He had a central line like Bryan's by that time. There weren't any veins that could handle the massive amounts of pain medication. Still, I didn't see how he looked.

His gaze had turned inward and the stare that accompanies the dying stared at me. But I didn't see it on one level.

I saw only Matt's spirit spread across the expanse. It was when he was in a room full of healthy, living children that I saw how far gone physically he really was.

Candlelight covered my thoughts the morning after Matt's last birthday. How did you do it, Lydia? What gave you the strength to release him?

"Who Will Come First?"

Matt's only time out of bed became bath time. I carried him to the warm bath and lay his head on one of those airplane travel pillows. His arms floated by his side as I poured water from a yellow plastic hospital picture over his thinning hair. I lay his head back on the pillow and poured more water over his body. We stayed until he grew too tired or the water grew too cold.

The gray travel pillow began to lose air. As nights passed, the pillow became more unusable with each bathing. The day came when Matt no longer could make it to the tub. It was the same day the pillow no longer held air. We get what we need until we don't need it anymore.

I moved the candle into the bedroom. How did you do it, Lydia?

One afternoon Matt and I were watching cartoons. We held hands in our silence. Matt said, "Herod is the goddess of wind and the goddess of love."

I knew Herod was neither, but the dementia had cast a long shadow by this point. I said, "Oh really."

He said, "Yeah. Who do you think will come first?"

I said, "I don't know. Maybe Mercury will come first. Who knows? Maybe Mama."

His voice was strong and sure. "Mama will come first," Matt immediately said.

We settled back into silence.

A few weeks later we were just days away. Donna was a regular visitor. The morphine patches increased and the injections in his central line became more regular. She couldn't understand how or why Matt was still alive. I knew, but I couldn't tell her.

Be it right or wrong I had enveloped my life into his. On a deep emotional level I had to confront the misconception that Matt's death was my death. No matter how much I intellectually disagreed with such an absurdity, the reality was I truly believed that when he died there was nothing left of me, or for me. When this was finished, I was finished.

The flame of the candle illuminated the night, no longer the morning. I asked Matt the day before he died, "When do you want to die?" He kept his eyes closed. He whispered, "I want to die when you die."

It was not love I needed to let go of; it was love I needed to let go into. Lydia left me with the key. It was in her eyes the last time her eyes opened. The culmination of the covenant was near.

"He Will Guide Us Safely."

I thought we would have one more day. At two in the morning he woke in pain. I medicated him, changed the bandages on his bedsores, and watched as he returned to sleep. I knew it was soon when my watch would end, but I thought there would be another day. Perhaps there is always a thought of one more day.

His breathing was soft. He lay on his back. I held his left hand in mine. I relived our first day together not thinking this was our last. It was his left hand that curled my finger in the intensive care the day of his birth when I said, "Hello, this is Papa. And I love you."

Thirteen years, one month and six days later I held the same hand. He was more unconscious than asleep. In the same cadence, into the same ear, holding the same fingers I said, "Hello, this is Papa. And I still love you."

The child I could not *not* love still lived where no one else could. I did everything in my power not to close off from him, as if that was even an option.

Matt woke in the morning. We watched television, holding hands. He looked up at the ceiling and said, "What did he say?"

"Who, Matt, what did who say?"

"The man." Matt's agitation grew. "What did the man say?"

"I don't know. What man?" I said.

"The African American man. What did he say?"

"Matt, I don't know. Who is he?"

He paused, eyes open and looking straight ahead. "He says he's the boatman."

"The boatman?" Then I remembered the Boatman in Greek Mythology, the one who takes people over the River Styx, across death into the underworld.

I said, "What does the Boatman say, Matt?"

Matt listened. "He said he will guide us safely."

He paused again before saying, "But I don't know."

I said, "No, Matt. You can trust the Boatman. He will guide us safely. Trust the Boatman, Matt."

Still, I thought we had one more day. Still, as much as I wanted to let go, I couldn't.

I lay down beside Matt at seven thirty that evening. I had been up since two in the morning and I needed a nap. I placed my hand in his and went to sleep.

The Covenant and the Goddess of Wind

I wanted to go the distance. Lingering in every act I took over the years was the deep desire to be there for Matt when he died.

To go the distance meant I would usher him into Lydia's love. I was to stand as I promised on this side, walking as far as I could into the length and width of finiteness. I thought she and I would meet where the Boatman docked and I would gently wave good-bye from spirit to Spirit. I had the vision of resting softly by his bed like I did with Lydia. It would be tender, priceless and unforgettable. His breath would change, just like Lydia's. He would look in my eyes one last time, just like Lydia. My child, my teacher, would impart in the ultimate moment where eternity lifts the veiled passage, and for one brief second I would again glimpse into Dream, and we would know each other as Spirit can only know.

It was the promise of continuity I yearned for, some remnant of the covenant between us that might be left behind for me, a timeless token I might hold when I could no longer hold him. All those years I thought if I can just go the distance, there would be something that I would be given to enable me to live when he died. More than anything I wanted to be awake – spiritually, mentally, emotionally and physically awake for the moment Matt woke within the realm, next to Lydia.

The last hour of my son's life I slept. I missed the last hour of Matt's life.

I don't remember the storm outside. It must have started after I fell asleep. But at eight-thirty in the dark of night a burst of wind crashed against the bedroom window. I jerked straight up, still holding Matt's hand; I turned to him fully awake from a deep sleep. Matt had two breaths left.

Matt's breaths were soft, barely rising, gently falling. I lay paralyzed next to two soft breaths.

I went into an emotional meltdown. It was not soft, far from gentle. I was hysterical. I didn't try to revive him, but I begged for him to come back. I leapt to my feet pacing the room, crying uncontrollably.

There was an indefinable implosion of my spirit. Matt's spirit was undetectable in my chaos and panic. It was the antithesis of all I had hoped. One hour of sleep woke into nightmare.

There was no stillness in my movement. And without stillness I was unable to follow, to enter, to exit, to be once again in the layer that all layers lie within. I missed it.

The wind only warned me of his leaving. It left me in the room, without passage.

"Herod is the goddess of wind. Herod is the goddess of love.... Who will come first? Mama will come first."

The wind woke me. Lydia came first. Herod may have been the Goddess of Wind, but Lydia came first.

He had to die in my sleep. I know. It was the only way Matt and I could untwine spirits enough to break time's grip. Just as I convinced Lydia to come home the night Bryan died, I had to sleep. I was unable to let go and it was the only way. But the mind isn't the heart. I understood. I even knew. But the mind isn't the heart.

I called Donna, the hospice nurse. I combed his hair, stroked his cheek as it grew cold, and cried. Over and over asking him to forgive me for not going the distance.

Memory's Mist

Matt's body stayed in the room of his death. Family and friends came to say good-bye. My father entered the house. He walked down the short hallway and into the room. He stood at the end of the bed when I approached the doorway. I looked at my father looking at my son. The room was full. I asked him if he wanted some time alone. He nodded and I left the house for a walk.

There must be some kind of guidance system within loss. I was simply putting one foot in front of the other on that crisp November morning, but my steps took me to the pier at White Rock Lake. I did not consciously go there, but there I was at the spot where Lydia and I shared an ordinary moment under an extraordinary circumstance. I had returned to the place she said, "Don't let him suffer."

The cool air matched the moment three years earlier. "Don't let him forget me," she said that day.

Matt never forgot her. The wooden pier rested underneath my bones. The sun was gentle. The sky blue.

Sitting alone for the first time left a surreal signature of what was, what isn't and what never will be. I wanted to feel Lydia, Matt and Bryan again, but I only felt the aloneness.

Stretched out over White Rock Lake was a mist of memory dancing over water I could not walk.

~ 166 ~

Ash to Ash

Several months before Matt's death we talked about what to do with his body. I picked an ordinary moment for the discussion because I didn't want it to feel like it was any different from any other conversation. Between baseball scores and hash browns in our morning routine I asked Matt what he wanted to do. Matt had two experiences – Bryan's casket in earth and his mother's ash on ocean. He said he would like to be cremated and his ashes spread like Mama's.

I then asked Matt about Bryan. I wanted to exhume Bryan's body and have him cremated too if Matt didn't have any objections. I knew it was not a rational desire. Death is death. Spirit is spirit and it really didn't matter on one level, but for me it was the feeling that Bryan would not be a part of the whole experience if I left him there and my memory of Matt and Lydia were over the Pacific. Mentally it didn't make any difference. Spiritually it didn't make any difference. Emotionally, it made a difference.

I said, "Matt, I'd like to take Bryan's body out of his grave and spread his ashes, too. Would you mind if I spread Bryan's ashes, too?"

Matt said, "Naw, just don't spread them on the same side of the boat."

The same funeral director that took Lydia's body took Matt's. This time I followed her. Several months before Matt died I asked her if I could cremate Matt's body myself. I wanted to be there. He was my son.

Needless to say, it was an uncommon request, but she found a mortuary with a crematory that would let me be there. It was about fifty miles outside of Dallas, east.

We put Matt's body in the back of her Suburban. I followed in my car. She drove the speed limit in the fast lane annoying everyone that passed us. I ignored the honking and stares. The mortician met us outside the small brick building. I took note of the smoke stack as I carried my child's body inside. He was a kind and thoughtful man. He was careful to see what I desired. My only desire was to go the distance.

Matt's feeble bones and skin were wrapped in a white sheet. I wanted only his nakedness to touch fire, but the man said it was standard for the body to be wrapped. I was so grateful for his kindness that I did not argue.

I lifted Matt's body into the oven and closed the door slowly. Flames made the only sound.

I opened the door and swept the bones and ash of my child into a container. We took a few steps to the crusher. He asked if I wanted him to pour the remains into the machine. I was his father.

I said, "No, I want to do it."

All those times I said to Matt, "It's an honor and a privilege to be your father," encircled me. It was my honor, my privilege, to finish what Lydia and I began.

It was eleven at night when I left with Matt's ashes. A cardboard box sat on the seat next to me. The highway was empty. I played the tape that Lydia listened to in her last days. The skyline of Dallas grew in the nearing distance.

A peace swept over me. The solitude of that moment moved me to stillness. There was an equilibrium that held me in the multi-layered instant. Life stretched in all directions. Present tense linked the unfolding of present tense like the steep slopes of a fjord links sea to sea.

It was while I was driving home that the present expanded to meet Moment, where Spirit intertwines with past, present and future. Just hours before, when I poured his ash into the bag, into the box, and into the car, I poured me into my stillness.

The covenant Lydia and I made was now finished. The sting of Matt's last hour was settling into its own unfolding. Only Lydia could have known what I felt as I rested in the space between light and dark. Lydia and I finished what needed finishing. Now it was up to me to finish the rest.

A Rite of Passage

Where does the death of another settle in the living?

Matt died on November 10, 1995. I decided to spread my children's ashes on February 28, the day Lydia died. The three months between was a period of closing.

Matt's funeral was not in a church. We had the ceremony in a beautiful room at the botanical gardens. His sixth grade class, now in seventh, sang several songs. A large picture of Matt in his healthier days sat on an easel. It was a very nice ceremony with many beautiful words filled with tender emotion.

Loss is a solitary path for me. I wish I could find comfort in collective sorrow, but it has never been my nature to do so. Kahlil Gibran in *The Broken Wings* describes it better than I. He wrote, "Solitude has soft, silky hands, but with strong fingers it grasps the heart and makes it ache with sorrow. Solitude is the ally of sorrow as well as a companion of spiritual exaltation."

As soon as the funeral was over I left. It was more than I could bear.

Bryan's death never settled easily within me. I was so overwhelmed in that period of life and the journey of stillness was embryonic in nature. I did not do the letting go of Bryan very well. His moment of death I missed. His room was empty on his last exhale. And at his funeral I was too consumed with Matt's state to fully experience and express my own. Bryan's eight and half months of life did not easily slide into a place of peace for me.

The stillness Lydia and I experienced in the last months of her life added to the expanse we were able to open. We spent many hours finding mutual ease. We were able to touch layer within layer on her way into death. I did not realize the extent of Lydia's wisdom until the wind swept through Matt's last two breaths. It was after that when all those late night conversations we shared settled into context. And that settled me. The softness of Lydia's last breath and the healing experience of spreading her ashes with Matt rested gently within me.

Now, where was Matt to settle within me?

Matt and I did not share years, months or even days. We shared something far more. We shared moments. But as much as I tried to let go, to match my breath to his, it was impossible. My inability to let go was what obstructed my deep desire to gently usher him into death.

I knew better. I just couldn't do better. I held him too tightly and the only way he could go gently was for me to sleep. Lydia warned me, but no matter what I did to heed her warnings there was this part of me that simply could not let go of him. And she had no choice but to come as she did. Matt could not have left any other way. Matt's death was soft and gentle. I don't live in regret over what isn't, or wasn't. What is, is.

However, Matt's moment of death was the most painful experience I have ever touched. It was cold, without heart and crushingly lonely.

Yet, the fulfillment of settling into Matt's death came on the ride back from the crematory. It synchronized me and gave me the congruency to move into the next rite of passage – the spreading of his ashes.

It also gave me another gift. If I could find equilibrium within my passages with Matt through what I thought I had missed, then there may be a chance to settle the unsettledness with Bryan.

Nothing is ever lost, only temporarily misplaced.

A Mendocino Storm

It is difficult to ride an untamed mind. My job was finished, both as a father and as an employee. I had no place to be, nowhere to go except to spread my children's ashes in three months time on the date of Lydia's death. I had three months to find some reason to keep living.

Dr. Viktor Frankl's book, *Man's Search for Meaning*, speaks of what kept Holocaust survivors alive. There was something beyond them that drew them from one moment to the next. There was a loved one they hoped was waiting, or someone or something that lifted them out of the abyss into hope.

A friend once told me she thought the best definition of the word spiritual was *what gives meaning*. My spirit searched for meaning and there was none I could find after the moment ash fell to sea.

I emptied the house, put a lifetime into a storage unit and left Dallas. The long journey back to California offered a different emptiness while an untamed mind rested on a catalogue of memories. The cold winter on the windscreen reflected the cold winter in my head. Miles under wheels, centuries under mind and meaning under Spirit fueled the passage of highways and back roads. Matt and Bryan's ashes, like Lydia's once were, sat beside me.

I stopped by Mendocino on my way to San Francisco. Even in the early '80s I was drawn to Mendocino, but Lydia and I never made it up there, which was a plus for stopping this time. I wanted to land where I could unpack a life and see what was left. I didn't want to be in San Francisco. I needed somewhere I had never been before. Mendocino was nestled in winter. The rainy season in Northern California was in full swing.

I entered from the north through winding two-lane roads. Huge redwoods and wild forest foliage pressed on both sides of the enclosed pavement. On more than one occasion I passed fallen trees that had to be cut to clear the road. The sky was pregnant with rain and I moved slowly around the blind bends that guarded the coastline.

I entered Fort Bragg, a town about seven miles north of Mendocino. Fort Bragg was blanketed by rain. The commercial fishing boats and logging community seemed stationary, Its streets uninhabited. I wandered the few streets of Mendocino between gusts of wind and sideways rainfall. It didn't feel like it was the place I was looking for – even though I had no idea what that was – I thought this wasn't it.

The street ended into a gravel parking lot. I walked to the rocks that stood between land and ocean. I curled up in my coat and sat on a rock near the raging sea, the same sea that was to be the grave of my children.

The Pacific Ocean was untamed and untamable. The surging waves slammed the massive stones sending a stream of spray into the cold hard wind. Saltwater dripped down my glasses, but without the protection my eyes would surely have been battered. The cold pellets of sea hurt as they hit my cheeks.

A wave snuck up on the rocky cliff and deluged the shore with a fiery power. Nothing could hold her, hold her back or hold on to her as she crashed again and again against the rock, against me.

It was then I knew I would move to Mendocino. She matched me. She spoke the language that spoke me. I was under the spell of her power, her unrelenting strength and her defiance. The Pacific's untamable spirit drew me into her. Between land and sea I was mirrored. She knew me and I knew her.

I cried and curled into the cold wind. The sea, ancient and wise, gave me the gift of matching seawater with salty tears, sea air with breath and Spirit with spirit.

When the sun shines over Mendocino it is stunning, but it was her understanding of sorrow that welcomed and embraced me that afternoon.

I continued on to San Francisco knowing I would return to where Mendocino presses against the Pacific and I would embark on my own search for meaning.

The Men on the Bridge

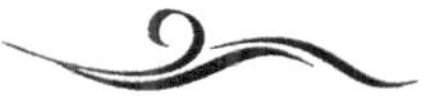

I stayed with Alan down in San Francisco. Alan was a parishioner in the Baptist church I ministered when Matt was born thirteen years earlier. He was the first person I called when Lydia had the seizures. He was the first one I called when we were in Colorado and got the news of their infections. He was the one we stayed with when we traveled through San Francisco. He knew Lydia before she was infected and walked with us through the years. Now he walked with me through the wait.

Alan's soft heart holds a wide berth. I have always been able to land within his kindness in any condition and under any circumstance. Alan opened more than his home to me.

I traveled those weeks in wait going back to the places that gave testament to Lydia and our children. I drove by apartments we rented, the seminary I attended, hospitals where Lydia worked and the hospital where Matt was born. I sat on beaches where Lydia and I spent our hours. I walked through Golden Gate Park, through the botanical gardens, the museums, the memories. There wasn't one place Lydia and I went that I did not go.

The night before Lydia and I left San Francisco for Colorado we went to the Golden Gate Bridge. Under the piling nearest the city we had a long romantic kiss, a kiss good-bye to the city we loved. On my return, I had a Walkman that played the tape she listened to as she died. The brisk wind slid past concrete from sea to bay. I strolled amongst the tourists out to the place we said good-bye, leaned over the orange fence and looked down into the sea below.

I wanted to die. Meaning, spirit, life and death went to separate corners. I did not know which corner to choose.

Lydia used to work at St. Mary's Hospital in the psychiatric unit. This was where they took the people that jumped and didn't die. She told me of their stories. Later, I met a dear friend who used to be captain of the Coast Guard ship that picked up the jumpers in the Bay. He told me about the ones that didn't live.

It took me time to filter everything I experienced and re-experienced on the bridge. But one thing I was sure of – I wasn't going to jump that day. I had yet to finish my one last duty. My children's ashes kept me alive.

I started back to the car. Walking the other way was a man, weathered not by the sun and wind, but by the street. His thin hair was disheveled and his face was carved with deep lines. His mismatched pants, shirt and coat didn't fit. Tucked beneath his coat was a sack with two bottles of beer. His eyes met mine; neither one of us turned away. He didn't have a desperate look and neither did I. His eyes carried no pity or remorse. He was neither empty nor full. I knew where he was going and I would be the last one to stop him on that day. We both had this brief unspoken agreement to not let the other go unnoticed.

A highway police car stopped next to me. The electric window on the passenger's side slid down and I leaned closer to the car. He said, "Are you okay?"

We both knew what we meant. I said, "Yeah, I'm okay."

He headed slowly down the bridge and I kept a steady stroll down towards land. I looked back at the end of the bridge. The police car was stopped with its red lights flashing. A group of people gathered by the piling at the far end. I don't know if the man jumped. I didn't look down at the water. I turned from the bridge to the city. I kept his secret, just as he kept mine.

I returned to Alan's house. Alan was the only man I know that didn't have a remote control for his television. He had had the same television for the entire fifteen-some-odd years of my knowing him. It was tough to mindlessly channel-surf standing next to the television, but I was looking for anything to tame my untamed mind.

It was a typical surf – forty channels and nothing on. I passed the *Oprah Winfrey Show*. Just at that moment Oprah switched on a television set next to her on stage, and there was Lydia and Bryan.

The day before Bryan died we recorded her dressing his central line. It was our only recording of Bryan. We had been on so many news shows this must have been some extra footage, but I don't remember giving the tape to anyone. I don't even know what context for Oprah was using the video. There I was standing in Alan's living room alone watching my son's last day with my deceased wife while the ashes of our children sat in the corner.

It was about as surreal as it comes.

I was so washed out I wasn't even sure this was real. But there they were. Bryan's deep blue eyes stare at his mother as she clinically circles his central line with a sterile swab, just like we always did. At the end of the tape Lydia sits down in the rocking chair with Bryan across her chest. Her job as Bryan's nurse complete; she becomes his mother again. Bryan's lips press against Lydia's breast. When she holds Bryan against her she can no longer hold herself at bay. She softly says, "Turn it off. That's enough. Turn it off now."

I turned off the television and looked out of Alan's window. In the far distance the Pacific Ocean looked back at me. It is difficult to ride an untamed mind.

An Innocent Heart

I had planned to spread the ashes of our children alone. It is a natural tendency for me to travel experiences of that magnitude unaccompanied. No one asked to be there. I made it quite clear from the beginning that the funeral was the collective time. The ash of my children and the boat ride to their grave was my time.

In the interim between death and the spreading of ashes, I returned to Dallas to load up my belongings. I kept most of Matt's things because I knew from experience that loss has its own rhythm; one touch of a coat could draw me onto a path full of emotional and spiritual treasures. I made every effort to keep whatever potentially opened me deeper. I would not let go of anything until it let go of me.

Skip was still relatively healthy on my return, but the decline had already begun. My moving back to California made what time I had with him special.

His small one-bedroom apartment was close to downtown Dallas. It was on the second story. I climbed the stairs thinking of how long he would be able to navigate them.

Skip's apartment was a true reflection of him. It was furnished in "Early American garage sale." He could see what others couldn't. He always found beauty when I would just see a piece of junk. It was junk until Skip touched it. His small two rooms housed a collection of unique and intriguing objects, all perfectly placed. Pictures and ornaments, tastefully arranged. It was clear Skip was moving towards death. Neither one of us was shy in discussing the inevitable. Death didn't scare him; it was the declining health that lay ahead that troubled him. He was blessed with the gift of being able to truly empathize. He was no stranger to pain. When he said, "I understand," he was not just saying it.

Skip has traveled further into the dark than most. He has seen the worst, and yet he still had the ability to see beyond the worst. But his best quality is that he makes me laugh. His dark humor tore at no one. He never puts anyone down, including himself. The thought of Skip makes me smile.

Skip knew the path he was on. He had buried many friends along the way. He had buried his sister-in-law and two nephews. He was in the midst of Kaposi's sarcoma, a skin cancer that tears the body apart. He had already lost and regained his hair, lost and regained his voice. Lost and regained his spirit. He leaned into life just like he leaned on his cane. We both knew what lay ahead. Skip could not tolerate the drugs available like AZT or D4T. It made him sicker than he already was. It was just a matter of time.

His bed would ultimately end up on the living room floor. His friends put together a schedule of round the clock voluntary care ready for the time. Stairs would soon be no longer negotiable. Hospice loomed. Death by attrition awaited my brother in the months ahead, but life was still good as we sat in his living room and talked.

When I placed my life next to his I could see farther and clearer. His generous spirit reflected my selfishness. His forgiving nature revealed my judgment.

It was in Skip's world where I saw how small my world was. I saw my selfishness in wanting to spread the ashes alone. These were my children, but they were not mine. It was still hard for me to bring anyone into my final act as a father; the hardest person to allow in was Skip.

I knew Skip was dying. I knew what memory envelops. It was a monumental ask of myself to invite him into the experience, because I knew what a shared memory changes into when death happens. The spreading of their ashes was going to be hard enough, but to carry the memory of doing it with Skip after Skip died would overwhelmingly add to my loss.

Lydia and I built a wealth of memories. Photos, letters, late night conversations, trips…we poured every moment full of what would be left, but what I didn't know then was what we collected was not finished once we closed the scrapbooks.

Nothing is stationary, especially the past. Colors change. Texture reshapes and changes. The context of one single event seen in retrospect can unfold and reconstruct hidden layers of an entire history.

There was a picture of Lydia holding Matt over a single rose when he was a few months old. We were in Golden Gate Park at the Rose Garden. The air was cool. Matt had on the white hospital beanie he got from the intensive care. The day was just another day. But death unsealed the past, throwing it into the wind. I held that picture by candlelight the night after Matt had cried himself to sleep because his mother was dead. Now the picture had changed; it was more than Lydia, Matt and a big red rose. It became a question mark, a semi-colon, an ellipsis that slid into the void. The candlelight unleashed an existential mystery in me like Alice's fall into Wonderland. It was no longer just a photograph. It was an indictment on all that life had become.

I loved Skip. I just didn't know if I could love him enough to hold another memory that would one day reshape into something else. I just didn't know.

He never asked to share the experience of spreading Matt and Bryan's ashes, but I so deeply wanted an innocent heart on the boat with me.

I had left my heart open to Matt. If I closed it completely, if innocence stopped at his last breath, then I would have negated a special part of my son's gift of life.

I wanted Skip to be there. I wanted another shared memory regardless of what death does to memory.

Ultimately, Skip's former partner and Matt's dear friend, Don, joined us. My mother and father also took to the sea to take Matt and Bryan's ashes to Lydia's.

To invite others was an important crossroads for me. I was at a turning point that I wasn't consciously aware of. A friend in Mendocino gave me some very valuable advice. Sandy had her share of sorrows. Her stepson was killed in a motorcycle accident at the age of seventeen. A year later her daughter was diagnosed with cancer at the age of eighteen. After her daughter died, her husband was murdered. Sandy said to me, "Keep your finger in the middle of your heart and never let it close."

Had I chosen to spread the ashes alone my aloneness could have entrapped me. Because I was able to open just enough to let another in, I was able to widen my loss to a place where it was both collective and solitary in nature.

There were times in Mendocino when I would curl tightly into a fetal position, grip my chest and be completely unable to breathe. The impulse would come out of nowhere, but it usually occurred at home. A massive wave of sorrow would engulf me and I just had to ride it out. It would last for about three or four minutes, but it felt like an eternity of hell. I would remember Sandy's words, "Hold your finger in the middle of your heart and never let it close." I would try to do both and breathe at the same time. The moment would subside. My red face began to pale. My body relaxed and I would wipe the tears away. Every time I went through this involuntary convulsion of loss, every time I kept my heart from closing, I always, always walked away with an expanded heart. I opened just a little more and consequently I experienced the world more lovingly. Every contraction offered me an expansion.

Skip is still alive. He was within months of death when the new medication became available. It was a big decision for him as to whether he would go on the new protocol. He had tasted the treasures of death and it was hard to pull back into life, but a friend convinced him to stay.

I'm deeply grateful he did.

What if I had made my decision to spread the ashes alone because of the possibility of not being able to cope with the memory of Skip's death?

I could have missed two very important features on the day we joined ash to sea. The first would have been the loss of shared history. The second would have been an open and innocent heart.

The Cake of Ash

Bryan Caleb Allen, born May 13, 1985, died February 2, 1986. Lydia Ann Williams Allen, born June 21, 1953, died February 28, 1992. Matthew Benjamin Allen, born October 4, 1982, died November 10, 1995.

I wrote the names and dates of my family, sequenced not by the measure of birth but of death. Bryan died first, then Lydia, finally, Matt. Death, the final measurement of this plane of existence, was how I collect them into me, into this dream.

The tidal moon determined their length of stay, for when the ocean rose in the night the names disappeared. And I was once again left with memory.

I held the boxes of ash as I stood on the dock with my father, mother, brother and his partner, Don. Five different people holding five different memories of Matthew Benjamin Allen and Bryan Caleb Allen.

The day brought dark clouds, pelting rain and howling winds. No one with a touch of sanity would have ventured to sea that day. But it had to be *that* day. It was February 28, 1996, four years to the day Lydia died. I wanted, needed, to end my last act as a parent on the day their mother ended hers.

I was grateful the captain of the small commercial fishing boat I chartered for the event was still willing to go, even though we couldn't go far. He stopped short of the spot where Matt and I cruised out on a sunlit day to softly slide his mother into sea.

The swells were massive. The rain scissored sideways into our path and a fierce, angry wind slammed the boat.

The captain steadied the boat as best he could. We took turns holding the plastic bag filled with Matt's ash. The others huddled inside the enclosed cabin as one by one we reached into memory, lifted the ash and let the storm rip it away. The captain's assistant stayed close to each of us in case an unpredictable wave took one of us overboard. The assistant was in his mid-twenties, unshaved and fit for fishing. He was a creature of the sea and blended well with the beat up fishing trawler. He braced himself to the edge of the boat. His legs rose naturally with the wave and rhythmically gave way with the boat's sudden descent.

This man I'll never see again did something I'll never forget. When each of us left the glassed-in cabin into the storm with a plastic bag of ash, he took his hat off in reverence. In a thunderous storm he lowered his hat to his heart.

I was the last to spread the last of my son, Matt. I was true to my word. Just as I promised Matt, I spread Bryan's tiny remains on the other side.

I went back into the cab. A film of Bryan's ash covered my left hand. A film of Matt's ash spread across my right hand.

We wordlessly battled the storm back to shore. I sat at the table looking into the remains of my children with what remained of me.

It was not ash on hands. It was hands on ash. Their ash was a testimony of the ash I ultimately am, and ultimately will be.

Sri Nisargadatta Maharaj, in *I Am That*, articulates the experience better than I when he said, "Just as every drop of the ocean carries the taste of the ocean, so does every moment carry the taste of eternity."

I looked into my sons. I looked into me. I looked at the eternal cycle of life and death. The boat made it back to harbor. We each exited the boat with different memories. I was careful not to touch anything with the remaining ash on my fingers and palms. At first I didn't know what to do with my hands, with my children. But I knew it needed to be reverent, some act that honored the eternity of the moment.

I walked to the edge of the wooden pier and lay my soaked body across the planks. My hands hovered over an ocean. The clear Pacific took the ashes and left my hands behind. And the ashes that held me, held me no longer.

It was time to be alone. My father, mother, Skip and Don left. I sat in my car drenched from the storm. I pushed the tape in the machine. The flautist that played for Lydia as she died now played for me. The parking lot was empty. The waves crashed against the harbor break wall of jagged boulders.

Where Heaven Meets Earth

On nights, other than rowdy, Matt had a nightly routine. We would read a book. He would put a night mask over his eyes and through headphones he would listen to the sound of humpback whales. One night I asked him, "Have you figured out what they're saying yet?"

He smiled and said, "Not yet."

I would come back later after the tape ended, take off the headphones and watch him sleep within his soft, steady breath. He slept in a dream and I dreamed next to him in the quiet.

Matt loved the sea. He also loved dolphins. One reporter that interviewed him wanted to talk about God. Matt said, "Do you know what my God is?"

The reporter was taken back a bit. She asked, "What?"

"My God's a dolphin."

She said, "Oh, that's interesting. Why is your God a dolphin?"

Matt said, "Because my dad says I can have any God I want and I like dolphins."

My father and I stood at some distance from the camera. I saw the cringe on his face when he turned to me. I shrugged. I knew Matt's God wasn't a dolphin.

Matt's God was love. At that moment love just happened to look like a dolphin.

When Matt was three and he said, "When I die, Mickey's going to come get me and we're going to dance on the clouds," I knew Mickey would have met him at death if he died at three. When the Boatman said that he "would guide us safely" I knew the Boatman would meet him at death. When Matt said, "Herod is the goddess of love and the goddess of wind" and "Mama will come first," I knew the wind that tore through the room the night he died was Mama, and who knows what Herod was up to that night.

Matt met love whether it manifested as Mickey, the Boatman, a dolphin, Herod or Mama. Love was what Matt met and entered in death.

A few weeks before Matt died we talked about sharing life from different sides of the same shore. I said, "If you can, give a sign you're okay."

He said he would, but didn't know how.

I said, "How about I go to Monterey Aquarium and if you're okay ask three dolphins to jump out at sea?"

He said, "Okay. I'll have three dolphins jump."

The storm that consumed Matt and Bryan's ashes still pounded the California coast as I drove from San Francisco to Monterey. I drove slowly through redwoods and coastline. It was a hope against hope. I took my time because hope was all I had left.

Monterey, the place of memory, drew me. The street filled with honeymoon scenes, a carousel, Lydia and Matt in Mickey Mouse shirts, Matt and I going through the aquarium after spreading Lydia's ashes. And now I walked the street to the aquarium one last time looking for one last sign that Matt was okay.

The aquarium was sparsely occupied. It was a weekday and there were a couple of school classes that herded from exhibit to exhibit. The outdoor theater was completely empty. The storm gave my solitude cover.

The clouds were sky high and the sheets of rain left the ocean enough visibility. I sat on the concrete seat scanning the ocean for three dolphins.

Rabindranath Tagore, in *Gitanjali*, describes the moment perfectly. He writes:

"In the deep shadows of the rainy July,
with secret steps, thou walkest,
silent as night, eluding all watchers.

To-day the morning has closed its eyes,
Heedless of the insistent calls of the loud east wind,
And a thick veil has been drawn over the ever-wakeful blue sky.

The woodlands have hushed their songs,
And doors are all shut at every house.
Thou art the solitary wayfarer in this deserted street.

Oh my only friend, my best beloved,
The gates are open in my house-
Do not pass by like a dream."

An hour turned to two. It wasn't really the need to know Matt was okay. It was more than that. It was the need to know, to experience, some connection between one side of the shore to the other.

The cold rain showered me, two hours turned to three. What I wanted was a sign, not of Matt, but of me. Three hours stretched to four. No dolphins. I was looking for something to make sense. Foolishly, I believed at the time that if I could just see three dolphins jump, time was truly wedded to timelessness. Here was woven into there.

I was cold. Just three dolphins. Wet. Still no dolphins.

The rain eased; the clouds were empty. I, too, was empty where dolphins didn't jump and Matt did not pass by.

Part 2:
Healing in the AfterLoss

Who gets up early to discover the moment light begins?
Who finds us here, circling, bewildered, like atoms?
Who comes to a spring thirsty
And sees the moon reflected in it?
Who, like Jacob blind with grief and age,
Smells the shirt of his lost son
And can see again?

But don't be satisfied with stories, how things
Have gone with others.
Unfold your own myth…

Rumi, verses in Unfold Your Own Myth

The Unfolding of Me

I returned to Mendocino to unfold my own myth. So much had collected in the brevity of my years, only thirty-nine then. I did not know what I was to find, or unfold. It was on my walks by the ocean that opened me most. The Mendocino coastline is beauty in motion. My weariness sat in contrast with her vitality. The shoreline held the pieces of me together as no other could. Her vastness spanned the horizon yet she pressed against land, pressed against me. Above her was sky, equally vast. It was large enough to hold my sorrow yet close enough to hold me.

The wind painted its own portrait, and like the ocean and sky the currents of air changed daily, sometimes from hour to hour. A slight breeze might blow. On other moments the fierce Northern California winds would curl the trees and force me to retreat.

Wind played an important role in my life. Wind carried Lydia to Matt. Wind carried Matt from me. A powerful current slammed against a window and my son's spirit lifted beyond body, beyond childhood, beyond father and son.

I can't say I found comfort in the wind as I sat on the cliffs watching Nature's dance. I often felt immobile in its fluidity. But I was drawn to the shore nonetheless.

It was in the torrential winds that I sank deeper into the shore, waiting for the Boatman. When would it be my turn? I often wondered when I came back from that near-death experience in 1976 whether I came back at all.

Everything took on a different hue after I was forced to return. I didn't want to come back. It was not my first choice. I found myself back in my body, spirit wedded again to name. When I got out of the car I didn't know which dream I was in. It reminded me of Chuang Tzu's famous statement on dreaming about being a butterfly. He woke not knowing whether he was a butterfly dreaming of being a man or a man dreaming he was a butterfly.

The wind, her power to destroy, her power to heal, left me huddled cold against the crashing waves. My lungs filled with cold salt air and pushed out again. The wind became my breath as I could barely breathe on that shoreline.

The sun rested light on ocean and land. The land and its majestic cliffs rested under me. The wind that took my son also kept me in my body. It was the breath of the planet that joined me to the elements of body.

A year before Matt died I developed asthma. I couldn't breathe properly and I wasn't even aware of it. I was in a meeting with some healthcare professionals at Parkland Hospital. One of them was a respiratory therapist. After the meeting he said, "You've got asthma."

I was a bit shocked. "What do you mean?"

He said, "You can't finish a sentence without taking a breath. Why don't you come by my office and we'll test your lung capacity."

I didn't even know I couldn't breathe. I was so consumed with Matt's care that I didn't hear my body crying out that it was suffocating. I was smothering myself emotionally and physically.

Matt's breath was growing weaker and so was mine. Air crawled into my lungs. And I didn't even notice it.

On the cliffs of Mendocino the fierce wind reminded me to breathe. It forced me to live in my body, to take notice of the cold at the very least.

The coastline and Nature's dance also drew me into the unfolding of my own myth. It was time to turn around and look back to where I had just come. As long as one of my family was left, I had lived my days in pieces. Mendocino gave me the gift of time to wander my own borders.

At times, without warning, loss would overwhelm me. I would find myself utterly immobilized or only able to do the simplest of tasks. It could strike anywhere and at any time. A song on the radio would trigger my unfolding. A candle flame could send me back to the candlelit nights by Matt's bed. A box of cereal at the store could drop me into another layer. Loss brought everything into question. What once made sense no longer did.

I was no longer the me I was. I felt like a skinless spirit looking for something to hold me together. One friend came to my house after I'd been in Mendocino for several months. He said, "Some of us are really worried about you. You need to get back into life. What do you do all day?"

I said, "I don't know, but it takes me all day to do it."

I felt I was in slow motion in a very fast world.

My Mendocino time was not a break from life. It was a period where I watched the scenes of my loss play and replay me. It was an opportunity to be still and breathe the coastal winds – the same wind that will one day come for me.

Sound is But an Echo

Will I still be able to hear the rain in heaven?

The sweet sound of a Mendocino downpour surrounded me. The sheet of raindrops slid through the sky onto a redwood forest, and then cascaded down the branches like a waterfall. I listened to the symphony of sounds. The highest branches whispered the arrival of each drop. The collision of water and earth sparked a richer tonal hue to the singing forest. One drop would sound a puddle, another drop sounded the ancient old growth trunk that fell, perhaps a century ago, and still another drop sounded me. Drop after drop, sound after sound sang in the sea of trees. I joined the sound, but I was a foreigner to this cathedral to Nature's beauty and power. I was the only human there, made with the sound of flesh and bones.

Matt was never far; for Matt was the most recent, most powerful in my loss. I began to measure the unfolding distance by the density of memory. If the memory of Matt faded even slightly I would rush to the edge of my thought and reel in the pain and hurt as if it were my only boat. Loss was all I had left. Would Matt die if my grief died?

My steps in the rainforest, or rather forest of rain, soaked my hiking boots. The thin rivers of rainwater flowed over rock, dirt, grass, fallen limbs and leaves. The sound of rivers, rivers in the sky, rivers through the branches, rivers under my feet, pressed my thoughts against the Boatman. "He will guide us safely," said the Boatman to Matt. It was the "us" that left me partly on shore, partly in the boat. It was the sound Matt heard and I didn't that I listened for in the forest.

"The movement of sound is not sound, but an echo," said the late Indian sage, Sri Nisargadatta Maharaj, in I Am That. The rain echoed. My heart echoed.

My life was lived in relation to other. But somewhere between the echo of the rain landing and the echo of me there was a vast chasm — silent, full, empty.

I had never been so alone. I felt hollow without him.

Loss spread time like a shroud of memories over an extremely feeble present tense.

The cold winter rain that had me curled under a coat wove me into the time Matt and I were huddled together in another storm. Yet in that storm we were safe and warm inside our home. We snuggled, bursting with excitement over the claps of thunder outside our window. We laughed each time the sky lit and another streak of lightning crossed the window in our first "rowdy night."

The sheets of rain cut the sky outside that very first night, just like the forest rain cut the sky above me that afternoon. A house, a home, separated Matt and me from the heavy downpour. Now thick branches broke the rain's fall before they fell on me.

I did not feel safe. I had no boundary to lean against, to glide my fingers across the darkness. There were no markers to measure meaning. I woke no longer needing to feed my child, prepare his medicine and start the day. I slept, no longer listening for him in the other room.

A brown fallen leaf lay inches from my boot. The extent of its life and the age of its death were unknown to me. But if it were not soaked in rain it would have been coarse and brittle. Instead the leaf felt soft, pliable and willing. I placed the leaf in the forming pool, close to the outlet that trickled down a newly shaped stream. It drifted in the pool for a time. I thought it was about to descend into the stream, but it got caught on small twig. I don't know which drop it was that collected in the cloud. I don't know when it left the sky to fall. I did not see it enter the forest and whether it took its time sliding from branch to branch or whether it made it directly from sky to earth. But I did see the single drop land. It exploded right on the edge of the twig and pushed free the old brown leaf. The current swept my companion into the stream. I rose to my feet to follow at a distance, keeping my eye on her. She joined other leaves in the stronger current, but I knew which leaf I'd touched. My eyes never left her. For a moment she fell still again. The edge of the stream gripped her. While other leaves continued on, she waited as the current beneath her slowly forced the muddy shore to let her go. I watched without interference as she rounded the makeshift corner and entered the creek that became a river. She sped down the river's flow to a sea miles away. And just like Matt, a brown leaf left me with only memory; the moment was gone, just the echo remained.

The Taoists have a concept called the Mysterious Pass. It is not a place. They say it is not found outside the body, but it is not of the body. The Mysterious Pass is the place, or state, that embraces the interweaving of both heaven and earth. It is the passage between the two. Maybe the Mysterious Pass is the passage between sound and echo.

A brown lifeless leaf caught in a torrential downpour in the middle of a forest of rain was my lens of Spirit. Its travels taught me the sacred simplicity of grief's gift.

My soul turned in the direction of the Mysterious Pass and on a journey. There was nothing that could not teach me. I had lost my greatest teacher – my son Matt, but another teaching had commenced.

Now It Is Time to Remember

Years before Matt and Lydia died, around 1988, I briefly met with a Jungian therapist. He suggested I write down my dreams. In one of my dreams I was standing next to a wooden coffin in a cemetery surrounded by mountains. The coffin was open and it sat next to a hole in the ground. There was marker with a name on it, a name I did not know. Inside the coffin lay five relics. I picked up each one carefully and returned it with equal care to its original place in the coffin. My grandmother on my father's side entered the dream. She picked up one of the relics with frivolous curiosity. I became frantic, and took the relic from her. "Don't!" I said, "You have to put it back exactly as it was." With reverence I tenderly returned the relic to its rightful place. Then I awoke. At the time I did not understand the dream.

In 1991, I was given the opportunity through The National Commission on AIDS to go to the International Conference on AIDS in Florence, Italy. I had never been to the heart of the European continent so I decided to leave a few weeks early, rent a car and tool around a bit before heading to Florence. I decided to fly into Zurich. I really wanted to experience the Swiss Alps. Since I was a small child the Alps was on my list of "something I must experience before I die."

I booked a ticket to Zurich to arrive three weeks before the conference. My plan was to get in the car and just drive, with no destination other than ultimately to drift down to Italy and be there on time for the conference.

During that period of my life part of my morning routine was to journal after my reflections. On this particular morning I wrote that I knew something was around the corner.

As I got up from the living room couch a wind blew through me. I now know the taste of such a wind, but at the time I only knew it stopped me in my tracks. The near-death experience of 1976 and the dream of 1988 melded into that. The words layered deep within thought rose within. It said, "Now it is time to remember."

I sat back on the couch and entered into the experience of death that I had avoided for fifteen years. The memories of what happened when I died that night in '76 flooded back. I remembered how my spirit felt as if it was hurtling through an expanse. There was no white light, no filmic replay of scenes from my life, no tender reunion with past relatives or calming words of comfort. I was sucked up in a torrent and dropped on a gentle, lapping seashore.

Walking next to me was Jesus – at least that is who at the time I felt it to be. I couldn't "see" him as such. He wasn't the white bread Protestant version with blue eyes. It was much more just a very deep sense of his presence. I was twenty years old at that time and my spirit was clothed in a Christian context. I assumed whatever spirit sees it will see it in those terms, just like Matt saw the Boatman.

We were strolling at a leisurely pace. We communicated without words. It was mind to mind.

I felt the conversation was didactic in nature. I did most of the listening, or at least he did most of the talking. The only words I returned with were at the end he said, "It's time to go back now."

I was surprised. I said, "But I don't want to go back."

His demeanor was as gentle as his words. He said, "No, you have to go back now."

I woke and dislodged myself from the backseat floorboard. I left the crumpled wreckage, lit a cigarette and walked away with only a memory of our last words and a pure state of peace. And now, as I prepared for my journey to Europe, it was "time to remember." I was clueless as to what it meant.

My first thought was I was going to die. In my lateral thinking I assumed I would be somewhere in Europe crushed in a car and this time I wasn't coming back. Ordinarily, dying in a car crash would not have been a problem, but Matt and Lydia were still alive at the time and it was my role to be there for their deaths. The timing was off.

Nevertheless, there was an eerie peace that filled the days before my travels to Europe. I had dinner over at Phil's house. He was more than just a boss and I told him about the experience of a wind that brought these other moments into one. He listened as he always did, without judgment.

After dinner we left the mystical and moseyed into the practical. Phil and his wife, Carolyn, had been to Switzerland the year before. He pulled out one of his maps to show me some interesting spots. Phil mentioned the town of Brunnen, a small village nestled against Lake Lucerne. He said, "It's a nice place to stop for lunch. It has some beautiful mountains against the lake."

When he said Brunnen, I knew I had to go there. Later in the conversation I said, "Phil, I need to go to Brunnen."

Phil did his customary wisdom-laced smile. "Yeah, I could tell. Maybe Brunnen is where you'll find what you're looking for."

My father was equally empathetic. When I told my father about the breeze that blew through me and all of its layers, he said, "There is a man in Zurich you might be interested in meeting. He's in his nineties now, but when he was young he studied with Freud. Why don't you tell him everything you just told me? Maybe he'll have some insights into the dream."

I arrived in Zurich with an address and a phone number. My father had told him I was coming, but nothing more. Over a cup of coffee I told him about the near-death experience, the dream and the sense that I needed to go to Brunnen. He listened intently and then said, "Go to Grendenwald. In Grendenwald you will find yourself." He drew me a map of where the cemetery was in Grendenwald. I thanked him and we left each other's company.

I was willing to go wherever led. So, when he said go to Grendenwald, I went, even though Brunnen still beckoned.

I stayed the night in Grendenwald and walked through the cemetery the next morning. Immediately I knew it wasn't where I would, as he said, find myself. I hopped back in the car and started down a road. It didn't matter what road it was; it was more important that it was the road beneath my wheels. I had truly let go.

This road ended at a National Park deep in the Alps. Where the road ended, the footpath began. I walked, still willing to step into the unknown, but not knowing how. This path ended at a brook. The mountain range in the distance punctured a blue sky and the sound of the tumbling water felt like a deep dream. I pulled my journal out of my backpack and wrote, still basking in the mystery. I was surprised when I wrote, "Grendenwald was nice, but it is not Brunnen. Tomorrow I go to Brunnen."

On the autobahn the light reflected crisp green trees, clear skies, and a deep hue of blue-silhouetted mountains in the distance. The sign said the next exit was Brunnen. The only landmark from the highway I saw was the steeple of a church. My heart melted into a knowing. The steeple drew me as if we were both in a state of wait.

I didn't know the way to the church. I followed the steeple from road to road. The parking lot to the small white structure had only two other cars; one was leaving when I arrived. I stepped out of the car as if the lot were holy ground.

In the afternoon silence I went to the children's graves first. I stood before each marker looking for the name that rested next to a wooden coffin filled with relics that came to me in my dream. The name was the only clue I had to the possibility of finding myself.

The small cemetery only had one marker I could not see. An elderly woman was cleaning the leaves off the grave in the far left corner of the adult section. At the far right corner was another grave. I stood before the mound of fresh upturned dirt that had yet to settle. The tombstone had a name, not the name I looked for, and carved under the name was the year – 1991.

I finished my unsuccessful search and sat on a white stone wall. I watched the woman caress the granite stone with a wet washcloth, as if tenderly bathing a child. I watched her and sank into my own memory of bathing Matt with the same tenderness. Before leaving I decided to go to the bathroom. I assumed there was one in the church so I went inside. Jonah had a whale. Jacob had a ladder. I had a vestibule in a Catholic church in the small town of Brunnen, Switzerland.

I had only been in a Catholic church once before. When I was twelve Skip convinced me that we should duck out of our father's Protestant church and sneak into a Catholic mass. Skip, the adventurer, convinced me that I needed to see what the Catholics were up to. He said, "Just do everything I do." We entered the church and in the back there was a pool of water. He touched the water, bowed and with his fingers touched his forehead, heart, left shoulder and then the right shoulder. I followed suit, scared to death they would find out that we weren't Catholics and we would be burned at the stake.

In Brunnen, the church was empty, waiting. An air of sacredness, a still wind, resided in the 15th century church sparsely filled with wooden pews on each side. I touched the holy water and for the second time in this life did the sign of the cross in honor and respect. Slowly I walked down the middle aisle. Statues of the twelve disciples hovered in concrete enclaves on each side. In the front was the bare wooden altar. Behind the altar, impaled on a cross, was the Christian God, Jesus.

I stopped at the second row and slipped into the right side pew. Lowering the prayer bench, I knelt with folded hands and said within mind-to-mind, "You've brought me half way around the world, what is it you want?"

Tears flowed, as if someone caressed me in the same way the woman caressed the stone in the graveyard. A century of tears streamed in our silence. No words answered me.

But a thought came. Augustine, one of the early Church Fathers, had a mystical experience at his conversion to Christianity. He was sitting in a garden and over the fence children were playing a child's game, chanting the words, "take and read, take and read." Augustine picked up the Bible next to him and converted.

I pulled out a hymnal and randomly opened its pages. The page fell on a hymn in a language I didn't know. Swiss German words paralleled melodies and musical notes. I can no more read music as I can read Swiss German. The only thing I was able to decipher was that the subject matter of the hymn was the Eucharist – the Last Supper.

In the Last Supper, Jesus took the bread and wine, gave each to his disciples as a symbol of his body and blood. At the end of the ceremony, he spoke the words that are etched in every altar, "This do in remembrance of me."

My tears were spent by the time I looked at the altar. I remembered the wind that breezed through me in my living room and the words, now it is time to remember.

My spirit stilled in the stillness of the moment of an empty church. The calmness equaled the walk I took by a sea in my near-death experience.

My path had already unfolded Eastward for sanity's sake, and yet here I was in this mystical exchange squarely in a Christological context.

I was done with battles. I had had enough. At that point, whatever the path, I was willing.

The oddity was that I was not drawn to Christianity at all. In fact, the interchange was of a completely different nature. I was not asked by the Divine, or Spirit, or higher self or any other term that might define and confine the experience, to follow the Christian faith.

I was released from the gravitational pull to a belief that wasn't mine. The borders I erected after my near-death experience in order to find order and congruency disintegrated that day. I no longer lived in negation, no longer measured my peace, my anger, my forgiveness by a God of judgment. I was free to love again. I walked out of the church free to follow my path without living in relation to anything but love – that place beyond beginnings and endings.

I sat on the stone wall again. The elderly woman still caressed the granite marker that separated her from her beloved. At the other end of the cemetery, the fresh grave had visitors. A young couple tended to the earth between them and the one they loved. A white butterfly encircled me as I watched the graves being touched so tenderly.

The experience had time to settle. I was in no hurry. I got up from the wall, went to the car and drove away, never to return.

I decided to go to Brunnen's town center to see the lake Phil described. There wasn't really a need to go there I thought. I had already found everything I believed was on offer. But when I stepped onto the promenade that rested next to the calm waters of Lake Lucerne, I saw something remarkable.

I suppose there is a place in everyone that is special. For me, there was this picture of a beautiful lake surrounded by mountains. As a child, whenever I was sinking into my most aloneness this was where I went. The woodpile in the backyard was where I played. A lake nestled in mountains was where I slept. And now, in Brunnen, I saw it again. Every shape of the mountains, shade of color, curve of shore was exactly as it had been in my mind's eye. This inner sanctuary where I had always lived, was an actual place.

The next day I ventured on the footpaths of Mt. Rigi, a ferry ride across from Brunnen. The land beneath me felt familiar to the touch. The mountain air breathed me, filling my lungs again. The sun scattered light through ancient trees. I strolled the path slowly, remembering, still wondering what the dream, the coffin, the relics meant.

It may sound a bit strange that I didn't go back to the church when I left Brunnen the next day. It seemed senseless to reach for what I already possessed. And as of yet, I have not returned to Brunnen.

The road to Italy took me over more Alps. It was an unusual scene. I felt as if I had entered some secret passage to the top of the earth. I drove past melting snowcaps on a treeless terrain. The air was thin high above the tree line and the sun sculpted glistening waterfalls out of snow and rock. What made this portion of the journey even more surreal was that I only encountered two other cars, both heading in the opposite direction. And I didn't know exactly where the road was taking me, which made it even more exciting.

Then the dream's interpretation hit me. I realized that the relics were five major faith systems. The one my grandmother mishandled and which disturbed me so much was that of Christianity. When I said to her, "You have to put it back just the way you found it," in that frantic tone, it was what I did in Brunnen. I put Christianity back as I found it, without malice, with love. The anger was gone; even the need to forgive or be forgiven disappeared.

As I drove across the top of the world I pondered what the rest of the dream might mean. I thought that maybe it was a sign that I should study comparative religions and examine their commonalities rather than their differences. I wanted to experience the unity of all things as expressed in our limited vocabularies of Spirit.

I thought that I might go back to school, get a doctorate and teach. I was in a bit of a career crisis since all my theological training and my subsequent shift away left me with no productive career path. To put it succinctly, I had no career. But the thought of more education and teaching soon vanished for two reasons – I wasn't the best of students grade-wise and I enjoy academics about as much as I enjoy a root canal.

And what of the coffin? Perhaps it was to examine death through the various systems, again looking for unity and the common thread that weaves us all.

But the unity found within belief systems was still just a shadow. The event that reflected the path before me was not the accident in 1976, not the dream in 1988, nor the Brunnen sanctuary in 1991. I did not realize then that the common thread was the wind that blew as I rose from my living room couch before my trip to Brunnen. The wind merged the accident and the dream within the recesses of my past and Brunnen and the Italian Alps within the recesses of my future. The wind that blew through me was the event that dissolved cause and effect, beginning and ending. Why did Lydia get the transfusion? Why did they die and I didn't? I no longer needed to make sense of it all.

What if Moment has no past, no present, no future? Even memory was laid suspect rounding the waterfalls on top of the Italian Alps. Something different, deeper, underlies life and links Moment.

Time and Distance

Solitude had always been my refuge. But after Matt died solitude was a vehicle to something that resided deeper in the labyrinth. I still reached out to the world around me, but in small doses. Mendocino was long walks and from time to time, intimate conversations with people of depth.

Jim was just about to retire. His salt and pepper beard was long. His eyes were aged, as were the lines that crossed his cheeks and forehead. Jim liked to mosey. He had worked for the county as a building inspector, one year left. But his true love was when he and his wife, Ruth, made a living fishing. His smile creased the well-earned lines and his eyes twinkled brighter than usual when he spoke of the open sea.

Jim and I had coffee often. I was drawn to his wisdom. Some people take up a lot of space, far more than they need. But Jim was the kind of man that took only what he needed. It was easy sitting with him. His words appeared to be unconsciously measured by an artful minimalism. We were at a small coffee shop in Fort Bragg. I had been on the North Coast for about a year. Little, if any, was shifting. I had witnessed the waxing and waning of loss and knew its signs well. This dynamic of waxing and waning sorrow could happen in a second, a day, month or year, perhaps a lifetime. The brief explosions of pain were far easier. They rose out of nowhere and ambushed me without warning. They were sharp-edged lightning attacks, but they subsided more quickly. And the scars they left healed quicker. I likened the experience to living on a fault line. The small tremors were a release valve. And I would console myself that the "big one," the earthquake that could take me down for good, was kept at bay for another day.

The slow moving expanses of loss were scarier, more ominous in nature. It silently crept along in the back noise of life, slowly eroding from the edges until it made its way to the center. It seized me, not by brute force like the quick bursts, but by attrition.

The most difficult aspect of the slow waxing sorrow was my inability to stop it. I had long learned that anything I resist I become. The more I tried to avoid the pain, the more I was in pain.

Grief was more tangible when Matt was alive. It was the touch of his hand. The sound of a whale tape. The light switch at the close of a day. It was the nights by his bed watching him sleep. The clock would whisper on the bed-stand, but time, grief's greatest ally, still had flesh, bones, breath. There was still a voice that made sounds, echoes. I could speak words of love to him, and hear him in return.

But loss painted a different hue after Matt's death. He was the last of the three. No longer could I hide in the touch of another. Barren of refuge I walked and breathed Mendocino.

Both Jim and I like strong coffee. On this particular day my loss was of the slow kind. When we had sat down for a cup, my grief had already slowly curled to a crescendo. I was beyond weary with balancing Moment and memory on this thin tight rope of time.

I said to Jim, "I'm doing the best that I can. I don't know what else I can do. When is it going to end? When will this pain stop?"

Jim had both elbows resting on the table. He didn't move a muscle as his eyes steadied on mine. His voice had the tone of subdued strength. He said, "It's just going to take time and distance."

Time I knew. But distance?

Distance. It was one of my greatest motivators while they lived – to go the distance, to be there for Matt, for Lydia and Bryan as best I could.

Distance. It was what Buck couldn't go. He hung himself before he could go the distance. His words followed me daily – "I'm not going to make it."

The coastline was peaceful and inviting. After our conversation I began to study distance of a different kind. To go the distance evolved into opening into the depths beneath the surface. Distance was now what lay within me, not in front of me.

The unfolding of Moment meant that I had to confront the past, not just the parts that were warm and fuzzy, but the past I would rather avoid. I had to move through memories of when words said and deeds done were like razors and every part of me wanted to recoil. I had to see, to witness, my perceived failures and embrace the totality of me, good and bad, strong and weak, finite and infinite. My selfishness, insensitivities and just plain stupidity had to be reckoned with, with grace, under a healing light.

A friend once said, "If I'm afraid of the future, it's because I'm still afraid of the past."

Life is a package tour. It was not easy to embrace all the things I wish I had done differently. But it's part of the package.

Rose Petals on Ash

Birthdays and death days were occasions of deep intensity. They carried the slow moving sorrow that started two weeks before the date and culminated in the day itself.

During the weeks before an anniversary I entered an involuntary stillness. Life on the outside would go on, but inside I moved in a different rhythm. My internal motion slowed. I like to watch people walk by. Give me a good cup of coffee, a seat by a coffee shop window and a busy street and I'm in seventh heaven. In the weeks before each anniversary I balanced my time with walks along the edges of ocean and forest and coffee shops.

I liked going down to San Francisco during anniversary times for three reasons. First, the beauty of nature that lies in pockets of the city, where Lydia and I took refuge on many days, helped me touch memory. Second, Half Moon Bay, the burial waters, drew me to her shore for the rose ceremony. And third, coffee shops on densely populated streets gave energy to the weariness that loss took.

I watched people with hurried lives hurry by. It was pure voyeurism. But it had purpose. The days before the day of the rose ceremony I slowed. Grief drained most of the emotional and spiritual resources I had. Coffee shops reminded me that I was the one off kilter. The world was still turning with normal people living normal lives.

A woman in a business suit and briefcase passed the window. Tourists with tourist sweaters huddled close together, inching near the crosswalk with glances in all directions as if they were being stalked.

In a way they were. A beggar closed in and the father with the big new sweater with the Golden Gate Bridge plastered across the chest, first tried to ignore the straggly bearded man. The panhandler was a professional, however. The crosswalk light turned green before the family man had to respond and his brood briskly stepped out into the safety of the street.

The beggar's face remained emotionless. A potential meal ticket had got away, but another one was coming. I watched him. I watched them – the ones that collected at the corner waiting for the light to change. I saw him leave some alone and others he would approach without reproach. He was streetwise and street weary. His energy was low and I watched him pick his movements with unconscious care. The corner was unproductive for his trade and he left, leaving me something in return.

Students passed, the city kind. High school kids less innocent, but still in possession of youthful eyes. Yet these eyes didn't miss a beat. I thought of Matt, thirteen at death, as the coffee touched my lips. He would have been fourteen.

The times I felt most grateful were when I saw a father and a son. It was impulse, not forced or contrived. It gave me hope to see another man living such a beautiful dream. I breathed deeper, moved closer to the human race when a father touched the shoulder of his child, when a child eased into the touch and they walked away. But if I saw a parent treat a child with disrespect, I was undone. A slap or a scream shattered me like breaking glass.

Fourteen. The 4th of October. I finished the cup of coffee a long time before I rose from the window seat. As I touched the glass door and pulled it away from the street, I matched my step with the ones on the street, walked in their rhythm while hiding mine. It was a learned trait Lydia and I developed through many days of living in secret. We had learned to hide the hurt, the physical deterioration, the depletion of energy. Camouflaged, we stepped into the world around us and blended with a thin veil of normalcy. Out of habit, I stood at the corner with the others, looking just like them. The light changed. They went their way, and I mine, in search of three roses.

With each anniversary of birth or death, there was a rose, a single rose for that particular one. But on October 4th I bought three roses. It was not only the day Matt was born. It was the day that Lydia received the transfusion. It was the day Lydia, Matt and Bryan began to actively die. October 4th was my greatest gift, and greatest curse.

The florist shop had buckets of flowers near the door. I looked for three specific colored roses – lavender for Lydia, yellow for Bryan and red for Matt. Each rose was chosen for texture, fragrance, the curl of the petal, the strength of the stem, and the thorns. I ran the outer petals across my closed lips to feel their touch, lifted the blossom near my nose and shared a breath.

The final test was the touch of the thorns. Stroking the stem slowly my fingerprint pressed each thorn to see if it was strong, yet supple. The distance from one thorn to the next played a part as well. Distance always played a part, whether it be a thorn or time.

Half Moon Bay was calmer than the day of ash. The afternoon wind was still strong, but the sky was cloudless. The sea rose, curled and crashed with force against the boulders left by man to divide open ocean from harbor. It was out on these boulders that I walked with lavender, yellow and red memories. My steps across jagged rock reminded me of another walk I made daily across the dam in Brownwood. It was ironic that my steps across the boulders in Brownwood, where I thought I was to die, were an exercise in staying in the moment. My steps across the rocks at Half Moon Bay were an exercise of moving within the realm of Moment. One was to stay present; the other was to meld past, present and future through a rose petal and a memory.

Lavender came first. Then Yellow. Finally, Red.

Waves crashed hard against rock. The sea flew into the air and slid across the dark russet stones. I found a place close enough to release the petals into the ocean's body, but sheltered enough from her spray. It was important that each petal landed in the sea, just as the ash that released my hands had to merge with the water beneath me. The timing of release had to take into account the wave's approach, the salty wind…and the kiss.

The petal always came first. It was the rose petal that released memory, not the other way around. I never tried conjuring a memory and picking a petal. It would have been artificial.

I held the first lavender petal. Lydia's favorite color. The memory that collected was the one in her front yard, the laughter that wove us and the gift of her loving me. The petal touched my lips. I chose my moment carefully and let go of the memory with the petal's release. The wave took only seconds to swallow her.

The next petal was for her being the mother she was. An ordinary scene wrapped in lavender touched my lips. We were in Golden Gate Park. Lydia was breastfeeding Matt. The sun came out from behind a cloud and she shielded Matt's eyes with her hand. My lips touched the petal and another memory floated on the sea for a brief interval between waves and then disappeared.

The ordinary memories felt the richest both in texture and taste. I let what come, come. There was no order to memory, just as there is no order to loss. The heart traveled the twenty-four years we physically knew each other, intertwining petal, memory and kiss. The heart added other memories, beyond death, like the wind that came for Matt. Another kiss, another wave, another petal went to sea. Each petal was laced with deep gratitude. She was a remarkable person. Each kiss honored her life. Each wave joined us in Moment.

Yellow. Sunlight yellow. Bryan's rose, Bryan's memory traveled different. His eight and a half months collected sparse memories, even sparser happy ones. He never could hold his head up or crawl and that was what haunted me most. I read books to him, but his eyes were caught between the vagueness of dementia and the relentlessness of pain. I held him, but was never sure how much I held.

The horizon stretched over the ocean further than I could see. I held the first yellow petal and let memory lead me, for my mind landed first on what was lost, not gained. This ceremony's only requirement beyond a rose and a body of water was that each memory had to be of gratitude. With Bryan, with both the brevity and brutality of his life, I had to hold the petal longer, go deeper into the distance.

The petal finally touched my lips.

Out of the canary yellow petal came the gratitude of his waiting after he died. I tried not to let my mind skip over the fact that my first taste of gratitude for the life of Bryan was in the hour beyond death, but I did not linger there. I returned to the heart, to the kiss and the gift of Bryan being the first one to teach me what death means on this side of life. He was the one who showed me the true proportion of a soul. Holding his body as it grew cold, feeling the warmth of his spirit hold me, was my first taste of what leaves and what is left. Bryan lit a trail I was to lean into under many a candle as Lydia grew near death, and Matt slowly emptied. I kissed the petal, waited for the perfect time and watched the first yellow petal disappear.

The next memory was his deep blue eyes – ancient and wise, powerful, strong, piercing eyes that took no prisoners. I was undone daily by his silent words. His eyes spoke centuries; windows opened from the inside. I touched the second petal with humble gratitude that I was honored to hold the gaze of eyes such as his.

For Bryan, memory collected on what he gave me more that what we shared. The brevity of his life robbed us of park swings, homework and video games, but his stay was long enough to touch my soul in a way no other could have. Of all of them, I bowed the lowest to Bryan.

Red. The color of the heart. I brushed my finger along the thorns of Matt's rose. It was a while before I separated the first petal. There simply weren't enough petals for Matt, or enough thorns. My ache for Matt was fresher than the others. This was the first birthday that we could not physically share.

From the age of three, when we found out about the HIV, birthdays were the blessing's curse. Each celebration of life marked this day – the day there would be no more birthdays. I would laugh and play, take pictures of him blowing out the candles and joyfully tearing through his presents as if he knew how little time we truly had. Beneath the gaiety, however, there was this day.

Thorns cut deep. I lived the celebrations wondering if another birthday party would come again next year. Would we have one more year? For ten birthdays I tried to push away the inevitability that one day would be this day. Yet, this day was always lurking in the shadows.

Lydia and I had learned well how to pretend, but inevitably, between presents, a slice of cake, or pin the tail on the donkey, our eyes would meet and reflect this moment – the moment I would be holding a deep red rose in Half Moon Bay.

As I held the rose, brushing my finger along the thorns, it was Lydia I yearned to be sitting beside me, not Matt. Just like the days after his death, it was Lydia; only Lydia would understand what it was like to be holding more memories than petals.

I was careful to tear the first red petal at the bottom to ensure the whole petal would release into my fingers. The soft thickness and rich hue of red did not go unnoticed. I encircled her with my fingers and held her at eye level. The wind stole her fragrance, but left a memory. My lips lingered against her softness. I thanked Matt for being my teacher, for widening me by becoming flesh. I kissed the rose petal again and let her go.

The sea engulfed her too quickly. Red disappeared, joining lavender and yellow.

Memory.

Each red petal disappeared as soon as it touched the hungry sea. The stem was all that was left. Moment does not linger.

I was alone, not in loneliness, but in a healing solitude.

The weeks before waxed to their zenith. The rose ceremony acknowledged the pendulum's waning back to a life lived on the surface.

I walked the rocks back to sand, then to the car. Lightness and expanse rested within me. I had gone the distance, as far as I could go at that point in time. Deep calls to deep. Three roses unfolded in an ocean and unfolded me just a little more.

Glass Beach, Glass Steps

Just north of Fort Bragg is Glass Beach. On top of the sandy floor lay thousands of multi-colored pieces of glass, chips of smoothed green, burgundy and blue glass no bigger than a fingerprint, all silky to the touch.

Glass Beach was where they dumped the trash into the ocean back in the twenties and thirties. The tide would rise and take refuse into the sea. Over the years, the ocean returned our trash to shore and the glass had found another shape in the ocean's depths.

Glass Beach attracts people from all over the area. Artists gather pieces to use for collages and sculpture. There are places to sit and enjoy the majestic view and rocks for children to climb.

One day, as I walked along the beach, I watched some children bouncing from rock to sand searching for shiny pieces that caught their eye. Their excitement was reminiscent of an Easter egg hunt. A sister yelled at her brother, "I've found the perfect one!" Her younger brother intensified his search, timing his steps by the surging waves.

The mother, in her mid-thirties, watched her children. She was peaceful, easy in her slow movements. Her flowing sweater puddled around the middle of her jeans and hid her old t-shirt.

Her daughter ran up to her excitedly. The mother studied the rock as if interested, smiled and handed it back and off the child went. She crossed her arms in the cool breeze and slid her feet slowly one in front of the other over smooth glass.

She seemed to be looking elsewhere. With one eye on her children, the other eye wondered out to sea. I've seen the look before.

Another woman carried a bag close to her side. She may not have been an artist. She just reminded me of one. She blended with the beach, the glass and the ocean. She squatted down and ran her fingers across the bright, glassy surface. She picked one up for a closer look. Her study reminded me of how I looked at rose petals. When she caressed each piece, it was almost a dance. It wasn't in her eyes. I was not close enough to see her eyes. It was the stillness of her body. The way her shoulders rested with ease. It was the time she took to touch what had been discarded decades ago and what she saw it was to become. When she found just the right piece she eased the glass nugget into her bag.

I watched the artist at work. I watched the ocean at work. I watched what was at work in me.

I had been in Mendocino for about a year and half, inching my way back to life. I liked Glass Beach. Broken discarded glass, submerged in the deep, and resurfacing to share in the creativity of creation again reshaped, renewed, reusable.

The first time I saw Glass Beach I thought of the old beat up trucks pulling up to the beach and mounds of trash thrown on the shore. I thought of the waves pulling our debris down into the dark waters.

Now, a year and a half later and many trips to Glass Beach, my thoughts centered on how the glass returned – What current did it ride to find its way back? How were the rough edges smoothed?

It was rare that I would find myself alone on Glass Beach, so initially I didn't stay too long.

I was so depleted when I first arrived on the coast and Glass Beach was my constant gauge. I would measure me by what shape I found myself on that particular day.

Grief had a way of veiling me as much as revealing me. I needed something external I could touch to give me proportion. Like a child's height being measured on the doorsill, I needed something that could say I was there and now I'm here. Glass Beach was this for me.

Over a year had passed. The shaping of me had smoothed. I could sit on a rock closer to the sea, the glass and the people. The sound of children triumphantly shouting their latest find no longer pierced me. I enjoyed the mingling of sound with memory, even experiencing times when sound had no memory. The artist's bag was full. She collected the usables and left.

I wondered if there was anything left in me to use. In my unfolding it was a tenuous time. I didn't know what was truly left. It would be a large leap for me to enter the world again.

I traveled down to San Francisco and sat next to busy streets wondering if I could live there again, if there was a place for me in hard-soled shoes on concrete. Where did I belong? I truly questioned if I could ever rejoin the human race again. The thought frightened me and it cut both ways. I feared I would never resurface again and I was afraid I just might.

There was a seductive quality to grief. I defined myself by what I was, what happened. The protective clothing of sorrow lured me. I kept life at bay with my loss. No one could come too close. My sorrow unconsciously had become a weapon, passive to the eye, but powerful in its pushing away anything that might come too close. It was an invisible cloak that I wore under a smile and a joke.

There was another feature of loss that enclosed me – the fear of moving on. There came a time when what saved me had begun to kill me. I had come to the point where if I didn't move, I would stagnate.

And yet letting go felt like a betrayal. Lydia said, "Don't let him forget me." How could Matt forget his mother? Oddly, when Matt was close to death he asked me, "Do you think you will forget me?" How could I ever forget him?

When I was a young pastor in Pacifica there was a woman whose adult son had died around twenty years earlier. She was completely homebound. Few people entered her small apartment, a shrine to her long lost son. I went every week into the tomb of her beloved. She spoke of only two things – her son and her physical ailments, which in reality were one and the same. I remember in my youthfulness the empathy I felt for her listening to the same stories of sorrow, how she missed him, how saintly he was and what happened to her the day she got the call that he had died, sudden and tragically. That day was the last day of her life. She had submerged into his.

Memory must metamorphose. There was a point where, if I did not go on, I would forever be going back. I needed to confront the belief that to go forward meant I had to leave the past. I still had this self-shaped identity of being a husband whose wife had died, a father whose children had died, and a man in the midst of grief.

In my black and white thinking I thought moving on was moving away. But as stillness widened me I began to see this was false. Stillness brought me to another aspect of Moment. The constant of my being, who I am was not determined by who I was.

For many years I had avoided the question of what comes next. While they were still alive I knew the future held death so I had learned to live in the present tense cherishing all that was on offer while we still had days left. When the last of our shared days ended I didn't care about tomorrow. I was numb and it didn't really matter what came next.

A year and a half in Mendocino began to change me. I sat on Glass Beach with a future. I had not had one in such a long time. It felt strange, frightening. I had lived longer than my past could hold me, but I did not know if the future was a sustainable option.

Observing the ebb and flow of grief was still my meaning, but it was time for me to leave Mendocino. If I had stayed I would have created a shrine to my family and hidden under the sprawling stars and ocean sunsets. As appealing as that might have been, it would have been the end of me. True stillness resides in motion.

Heading East

Where was I to go now that freedom said it was time? I was forty years old, no family and no place in particular to be. I decided to go to Asia, for no reason at all.

I couldn't see myself staying in the States and I thought before I settle down I'd like to live in another culture. I had never been to Asia before, and never been out of the U.S. to live.

I found a job in Lampang, Thailand, teaching English at a small university. Everything fell into place in applying for the job so I figured that was the place.

I didn't have any friends who had been to Thailand. I was clueless as to what was there. I just had a sense that this was where I was to be. I could live simply on a teacher's salary, save my depleting cash and see a bit of Asia.

On a deeper level, however, it was an attempt to get back into life. I had harbored in Mendocino long enough to feel more than death. The beginnings of wanting to live again started to bud.

It was not as if I were going to Washington to a high-pressured job, or to a non-profit organization hustling to meet budgets and quality care. I wasn't ready for something like that. I wasn't sure if I would ever be. Here was a chance to dip my toes into the stream and see if there were crocodiles.

All that said, it wasn't really why I went. I went because there was an innate knowingness that was the grounded within the Unknown. I just felt drawn to Thailand.

I do not fear what lies ahead because I do not fear what lies within. And the best way to prepare for the next moment is to live fully in this one.

Just having nothing to lose – my real impulse for deciding to go to Asia – had reached another layer, richer and more aligned to freedom's true texture.

Life never turns out how I think it will. It was senseless for me to even to try to imagine what would happen in Thailand, but try I did. And I was wrong about everything except one premonition. And even that took its own course in its own way.

"We Come in Peace."

About thirty thousand people live in Lampang, Thailand, a little over two hundred of them being foreigners. The college I taught at was a private school. I was told before I left the U.S. that all Thais have studied English in junior and senior high school.

The first day of class only eight students out of thirty showed up. I thought "now this is my kinda school." The students looked back at me like someone would look at a monkey caged in the zoo, but with less interest.

I said, "How many of you have studied English?"

Silence. Not even a muscle moved anywhere on their collective bodies.

"English? Study?"

Nothing. Completely expressionless.

"High school?"

Blank. Nada. Zip.

If I were in a poker game, I would have folded right then and there.

I wrote the word English on the black board, turned to the class and smiled nervously into the void. All thoughts of lesson plans and creative role-playing drained to the ground like the sweat on my palms.

Later I was told, yes, they had studied English in high school, but from a Thai teacher, with a Thai accent. My diction was completely foreign, literally. And another teacher informed me that the complicated verb forms were probably a deterrent as well. Thais have a less complicated conjugation of verbs. Past tense, past participles and all those other kinds of verbs that try to put words to time don't exist in Thai. Smart people these Thais.

I stood before these eight blank faces for about fifteen minutes. I thought I might spread my arms out and like any good alien from another planet say, "We come in peace."

I was a big hit when I dismissed class sixteen minutes into our initial "exchange." I folded. They won.

As the semester progressed so did I. The gifts of these students were their kindness and patience. I definitely learned more than they did. I stepped into their culture with mine still entrenched. I learned that another's culture is just as sacred as another's heart. When cultures truly meet, they do so in a new language, uncommon to culture, but common to all cultures. It requires a language of the heart rather than past participles and prepositional phrases, and it speaks from an ancient place carved by centuries of interweaving people to people.

The final exam was a wonderful example of a clash of cultures. There is a collective spirit in Asian mores. What in the West would be considered cheating, in Thailand would be considered as helping your friend. The West glorifies self-propulsion and individual achievement. The Thais honor friendship and collective concern for each other.

Once I watched a group of students in the break. Two headed off to the cafeteria and returned with some snacks. It looked to be only enough for them. But without the others asking the two instinctively shared what they had with the others. It was as natural as sunlight resting on a leaf.

The teachers were told to teach as if in the West. Cheating was cheating. But I had long learned that I had entered their world. They had not entered mine. Helping was helping. We were told to drill the students with the consequences of "helping" their friends. Cheating would mean an automatic fail.

It was excruciating watching the four-hour final exam. All the English classes combined in the large auditorium. The foreign English teacher strolled the aisles. In the first hour there were a few sideways glances, but they were subtle and fairly benign. The second hour brought longer looks. And the friend "helping" conveniently twisted the paper for a better look. In the third hour, a few of the students handed in their exams and headed out into the day, leaving little pockets of students scattered across the room, still glancing at the roving teachers and their friend's paper. By the fourth hour, desperation had set in. Students craned over their friend's shoulders. I watched them until they looked up to see if I was looking and then I turned away.

Who was to say which way was best? East or West?

My only goal as a teacher in that one semester was to make learning English less painful. I had lost any expectation that they would be conversing in an extremely difficult language. All I wanted to do was to give them a positive experience so if one day they really wanted to learn English, they would think back to that odd American that didn't bust their chops.

Motorbikes and the Watercourse Way

Another way to describe my experience with Thai culture was its traffic. The road rules of Thailand were more a suggestion than a demand. I was taught in America that a red light meant stop. In Thailand, a red light meant it'd be a pretty good idea, depending on the traffic and just how long the light has been red.

Also, there was this mysterious "middle" lane on a two-lane highway. Cars hurtled from either direction in the middle of the road regardless of what was coming the other way. There was an unspoken understanding that the approaching cars would ease to the shoulder and this middle lane would suddenly appear. The passing vehicle would harmoniously move without flinching. No one seemed to flinch on the highways in Thailand.

Often I would drive around in the mountains outside Lampang on my motor scooter. There was something healing about cruising through the luscious forests that surrounded the town. These little scooters can get up to quite a clip. I was on a two-lane highway just outside the city, flying about fifty-five miles an hour. In the distance on this long stretch of road was one car. Then a truck started to pass in the "middle" lane. I thought "no problem, plenty of room." But then another car started to pass at the same time. Coming my way in parallel formation were two cars and one truck. I had about a meter of shoulder to play with and a ravine to my left. There was no time to slow down or turn, ninety kilometers of speed and about sixty seconds to make a decision.

Both cars and the truck didn't flinch, pause or retreat to offer me any room. I had no expectation they would. I really had only one course of action – to stay the course. The shoulder beneath my wheels was soft. Slight movement in any direction except forward would have dire consequences. I didn't slow down for fear of the bike making an uncertain movement. If I were going to die I would just as soon die at ninety kilometers as opposed to sixty.

I was remarkably calm. There is something about leaning into fate's inevitability that creates a feeling of peaceful resignation. Seconds slowed as they usually do under the increased speed of time. My life didn't pass in front of my eyes, but a couple of thoughts did. My mind settled oddly on relief. There was no grasping for another moment, no wanting just one more day, nothing, just a sense of "okay, whatever."

I looked up from the gravel as they drew nearer to see if there were any last minute adjustments I could possibly make. I measured the distance from my mirror to his. I did not look at the driver, the row of cars, the mountains or even the gravel. With three seconds to go all I looked at proximity of mirrors.

As we passed I didn't tighten. Strangely, my body sunk deeper into the seat and my hands softened around the handles. There was ease to my inhalation. And when we passed without incident, my exhale was like a long, peaceful sigh.

After it was over I thought, "those crazy idiots! I could have been killed!" I was still living in the States while my body was in Thailand.

I thought there was no rhyme or reason to any traffic laws in Thailand. But the traffic in Thailand has very defined laws, maybe they are unwritten, but they were there for all to see if they cared to look.

Once I stepped out of my boxed-in beliefs I began to see a different way of embracing traffic, and Thailand itself. The movement of cars and multitude of motor scooters through the streets and highways had an ebb and flow. In a water-like way, the collective rhythm of the road was at work. Thai drivers had this uncanny ability to move with the traffic as if it were a stream within a well-known current. And I realized that it was not individual cars or bikes that moved on the street. It was like a harmonic concert at every juncture. Thai drivers have this capacity to see the whole and move with it where I was taught to mark my space, calculate what I needed and act accordingly. The Thai way was to move with what is. The rules of the road widened me to see the whole scene unfolding in a natural flow, a natural law of traffic. There was a collective understanding. Of course the bike was going to enter the road with oncoming traffic and we will all move over to accommodate; of course there is a middle lane. What's the problem?

Where Does It Hurt?

I was still filtering my experiences through my grief. As I moved in time further from their deaths, I found an interesting dynamic I had unconsciously created in the filtering of life. I had codified and catalogued experience through the template of what was. Memory, which was a nurturing healer, was also the destroyer of present tense.

Thailand called into question my plethora of staid beliefs. And that called into question how I grieved and how most of my points of reference for my life were built and perpetuated in death's shadow, not death's light.

I knew Thailand was not to be a permanent home. My body didn't fit Thailand. I like to blend, meld into the scenery and this was not possible in Lampang. It was not unlike the years spent with Bryan, Lydia and Matt. My body, healthy and living, did not fit with theirs. It was a painful exclusion. Thailand felt that way for me. It was an external reminder that I still did not fit.

Lek was a Thai masseur. He was in his mid-thirties, slender, graceful, with high cheekbones. He was studying to be a lawyer when a car accident took his sight. He spoke a little English. I spoke less Thai. It was his hands that carried the language of wisdom.

Thai massage is not gentle, but there was a gentleness in his strength and power. He knew the limits of my body and harmonized his power to expand my muscles to their capacity without crossing the line.

There are a lot of odd contortions in Thai massage, some quite challenging. But I trusted him. He would turn my head and I relaxed my neck in his hands. Not an easy thing for me to do. Since my own car accident, my neck has never been able to sink into a natural state and it was a constant reminder that I walked away, and what I walked away with.

He moved his fingers across my legs. I closed my eyes, superficially matching his darkness. His power was not in the pressure that he ultimately applied. I found his power was in his search for what I held, blocked and had in one shape or another refused to relinquish.

The man without sight saw, with his fingers, a man who could see, but not very far.

My body held reference points. It was my first experience of just how much memory the body holds. My body and I had this unspoken truce. I asked for my body to get me from point A to point B and in return I'd do my best to treat it nicely.

It was the beginning of a very long road in finding harmony between body and soul. I made very, very small steps in Thailand in that direction. His weekly massages were a crucial element in my beginning to see that the reference point of my physicality was an intricate part of my moving through the grieving process. The body holds memory. And as I began to be aware of the body and point to where it hurts, I began to go deeper into opening the gift of grief.

Chiang Mai and Mountain Clouds

I went to Chiang Mai every weekend. Chiang Mai is ninety-nine kilometers from Lampang. I'd catch a bus for the two-hour trip.

If anyone wants to find God, sit in the front end of cross-country Thai bus. These drivers know no fear. I was told by another foreigner to sit close to the back. In case of an accident there is a better chance of surviving.

Rice paddies rested on the plains surrounded by luscious mountains on the way from Lampang to Chiang Mai. Postcard kind of stuff. From time to time there was a burned out bus languishing on the side of the road. Not in the postcard.

The heat, the cramped quarters, the middle lanes and the fearless drivers made the trip feel like an endurance test. Just when I thought I had had enough, enough had more.

Chiang Mai is the second largest city in Thailand, second only to Bangkok. It sits in a valley with mountain ranges in full view in either direction. However, the city lives closest to Doi Suthep, a beautiful testament to Nature.

Doi Suthep does not reach high. When I looked from the ground up the lush shades of green looked like stairs to the heavens. When my eyes started with the sky and descended it looked like a cascading waterfall of green streaming gently into the city.

The clouds that sit atop of Doi Suthep in the rainy seasons stretched effortlessly skyward. White vapor mountains moved slowly across the blue backdrop. Some rested on the shoulders of Doi Suthep for hours with no need to move at all. But sooner or later the breeze pushed the clouds over the city and the rains would wash the old streets, cleaning her shops, bars and temples.

Chiang Mai was a city of contrasts. Like any city anywhere in the world Chiang Mai had its seedy side. The traders traded everything while all the surface dwellers from other countries huddled in their desires for the best deals.

Chiang Mai also had a loving side. Beautiful people lived with honor and respect, genuine love and kindheartedness. This was the true world of the Thai people, but it was a hard world for a foreigner to penetrate.

My friend in San Francisco, Alan, was a cop in Oakland back in the early sixties. He shared with me his experience with the Berkeley student protests, their volatility and the underlying dynamic of people pressing in anger against each other. He said that when the line was drawn between the protesters and the police, the closer to the line drawn, the more hostile and radical the people were, both cop and protester. But the further from the epicenter, both the cops and protesters were more sane and humane, common folk not wanting to do harm, just wanting to live and be at peace.

My experience with Chiang Mai was a lot like that. The closer to the traders, both foreign and domestic, the more a culture of scarcity and greed dwelt. The further the distance from the tourist traps, the more real the people became. I had the good fortune of meeting some extremely wonderful Thai people, real families with great integrity and kindness.

When my bike broke down, a passing truck stopped. The driver tossed my bike in the back and took me to a station kilometers down the road. I was lost one day and a man with his young child spent a great deal of time to help me find my way. Many, many times my heart was renewed by the generous acts of the Thais.

On the other side of the ledger, I did not fit well with the traders, both sides of the trade. The energy of such a world depletes. It deadens the senses when anyone looks for what they can get rather than what they can give. The dullness behind the smiling eyes barely concealed the language of lethargic emptiness. The closer to the line where tourist and trader sought the spoils, the closer I felt the emptiness, theirs and mine.

This kind of emptiness, coupled with my inability to truly enter the inner recesses of the culture, reminded me once again that I was on the outside. Loss took me outside of the stream of America's collective. I did not feel I belonged on the streets of San Francisco any more than I felt I fit into the streets of Chiang Mai. One coffee shop was just like any coffee shop anywhere. People traveled by and I watched other lives live what I couldn't. Chiang Mai just put it more in my face, but I couldn't hide my loneliness and isolation in Chiang Mai like I could in San Francisco.

Also, in San Francisco, I dressed my moments in what was. My point of reference was death, memory, ashes out in the sea, cool winds that had the faint scent of the wind that took Matt.

I went to Thailand to move on, but found myself moving further away. I was still a stranger in a strange land in Chiang Mai, just as I was a stranger drinking coffee at Union Square in San Francisco.

I had decided at the end of the semester I was going to leave. I just didn't know where to.

East, West and In Between

Roland was passing through Chiang Mai. In Sydney, Roland had developed a writing school called The Writer's Studio. Once a year he would bring a group of Aussies to Thailand for an intensive writing workshop. In the next day or two the latest group was to arrive.

We talked for a long time. Shared interest was rare for me in Thailand. Roland and I were the same age, we both were interested in writing, and we were both passing through. I told him I was leaving in a month when the semester finished, but wasn't sure where I would go. Roland suggested Sydney. He spoke of the writing courses he did there and the beauty of the city. Roland was one of the best salespeople I've ever met because Roland didn't sell, he offered. He believed in his product and his low-key way of presenting it gave me room to consider the possibility of going down under.

He said, "We're going to have a welcome dinner for the writing group tomorrow night. Why don't you come along?"

I thought I might as well. What's it going to hurt?

Roland and I were to meet at his hotel, The Montri, the next night. The Montri Hotel sat next to Tha Phae Gate, the wall to the old city. Motorbikes and cars constantly stream by the four-story building.

I went into the semi-plush lobby with a book in hand to wait. I had already found out that Roland was punctually challenged.

I remember the moment I saw her. She sat on the couch in the lobby reading a newspaper with intermittent glances towards the hallway leading to the rooms. The waves of her long blonde hair stood in contrast in the sea of black hair of Thailand.

I sat in an upholstered chair in the same semi-circle of furniture around a glass coffee table, one eye on a book I wasn't reading and my good eye on her. She was mildly preoccupied. She rose and circled the couch on the right to pace between the back of the couch and the hotel desk. I watched her slim body, hidden beneath a flowing white blouse. I could tell she was waiting for somebody, probably a husband or lover by the look of her.

There was an old attraction at play. I kept my glances at a safe distance. I studied me studying her. My feelings felt rich and aged like a smooth wine, groomed by time. It wasn't a palpable desire or hunger that rose within me. It was a sinking into memory, still out of reach and vague, but memory nonetheless, that drew me to her.

I found her pacing cute. My soul hid in the shadows as she checked the clock and then turned again to the hallway with arms folded. Someone was late.

Roland strolled out into the lobby as if time had no meaning. As I rose and approached him, so did she.

Roland looked mildly surprised to see us both standing in front of him. I was more than surprised and pleasantly pleased. Roland introduced me to Rachel.

Rachel was coordinating the group of incoming Aussies. She was British by birth, but she had lived in Chiang Mai for the past eight years. Before that she lived in Hong Kong for five. As soon as she graduated from university in England she left her family on the outskirts of Bristol and headed east.

We shook hands, exchanged greetings and headed out the door to our respective motorbikes. Rachel had the idea of getting flowers for the arriving guests. Roland agreed and suggested she should go in the direction of the market and he would go to the restaurant since they were running a little behind schedule. He asked me, "Would you like to go with Rachel?"

Tough call.

Rachel led the way on her bike. The beat up old bike didn't have a backlight so it was easy to detect. She zipped through the traffic like water on water. I kept my eye on the thick blonde hair flowing out beneath her helmet.

On Charoen Prathet Road a row of florist shops sat open faced to the river that ran across the street. The rows of roses, birds of paradise, and all varieties of Thailand's color matched the beautiful fragrances that competed with the passing exhaust fumes.

Rachel pulled her bike to the curb and I followed. The market was vibrant and alive. The heat of day was forgotten in the coolness of night. It was alive with people wandering the streets from fruit markets, meat stands and small makeshift cookeries. The florist stands were at the end of the line.

Rachel spoke flowing Thai to the shopkeeper and the negotiations began. I watched as back and forth they smilingly bartered in a light lilt. I caught a word that was the mark of money. The saleswoman named a price. Rachel looked back in surprise and let out the traditional response of disbelief. It was part of the game. She studied the flower bouquet and shook her head no.

She looked at me and let out a slight laugh, closer to a chuckle. That's when Moment met memory. It was the laugh, short and light, where I caught the briefest of glimpses of that place between sound and echo.

It reminded me of an old folktale of a Taoist monk and a monastery bell. In ancient times, around 330 B.C.E. a boy of three was left at a monastery on the edge of Taishan, a sacred mountain in China. As the days passed the boy forgot the ones that left him and the old monks became his family.

At the age of six it became his job to light the morning candles leading up the bell tower, one candle for one step in the circular stone stairway. At the top of the small tower, every day the boy lit the last candle just as the sun rose from mountain to sky. As streams of sunlight embraced the candle, the boy pulled the rope and the rich tone of the ancient bell echoed in another day.

To the boy, the ritual became a job. And his heart went out with the ringing of the brass bell as it journeyed far beyond the monastery walls.

Time passed and the boy began to dream about what lay beyond those walls. At eighteen, he decided to leave the monastery to see the world. On his last day, he was so pre-occupied with his pending journey that he barely noticed the sound of the bell.

His travels led him in many directions, tasting life's many flavors. But as he grew old he began to return to the old ways. He settled in a hermitage far from the monastery of his youth, a small thatched hut deep in the forest.

He shared the woods with the spirits of the forest. Through the years the small hut started to become too small for his passage into timelessness. The spirits that visited him knew he was not long for this plane and knew he was troubled.

Spirit asked, "What is it boy? What troubles you? Death?"

The aged boy laughed. "No, it is not death that troubles me."

The spirits spoke among themselves and Spirit asked, "Do you feel sad that you have not attained enlightenment?"

The boy again laughed. "What is there to attain? No, it is not enlightenment that troubles me."

"Then what is it, boy?"

The boy touched the embers of the small fire with a stick. Small flickering sparks lightly ascended and disappeared in the dark.

"It is the ringing of the bell. The last time I heard the bell I did not hear it. Before I die I would like to hear the ringing of the bell."

The spirits whispered among themselves and Spirit spoke. "It is a long journey from here to there."

"Yes, I know. But the one thing I want most is to hear the echo of her sound once more."

"Why?" asked Spirit.

Another ember disappeared above the fire.

The boy said, "It will complete me."

Spirit blessed the boy and at the age of ninety-one the boy rose with everything he had left – just his sack, his walking stick and the memory of the bell. He started east, over the mountains.

A year passed. The embers of the boy's eyes were fading. The bones of his right hand curled the walking stick leaving a mark on both. Each day his steps grew him closer. Every morning, when the sunlight rose over the mountain, he listened for the echo that would lead him to the sound, but only memory guided his steps.

The monks did not remember him the night he arrived. No one that knew him was still alive. But when he told them of the ringing of the bell, how the sound of heaven and the echo of earth clothed a morning sky, how the wedding of candle and sunlight carried a deeper sound and how sound carried soul, they recognized the boy as one of them. The abbot said, "Would you like to ring the bell in the morning?"

The boy smiled and bowed. "It would be my greatest honor."

The boy did not sleep that night. He rose from his cot at four in the morning. As he sat in meditation his stillness passed from moment to Moment. Spirit met the boy there to wait.

He rose at the appointed time and stood at the bottom step. One step. One candle.

The long journey had wearied the boy. Another step. Another candle.

His legs, taut from the trek, were steady as he pressed his sandal against the uneven stone beneath him. Each candle lit the promise of reunion of echo and sound.

He touched the rope and gripped it with the callous hand that gripped the walking cane through all those mountain passes. He closed his eyes, took a deep breath and pulled the rope.

The vibration of the brass bell made his hands tremble. Sound kindled echo. Echo rekindled the boy. Across Moment they met again.

The sound of Rachel's laugh crossed Moment. The turn of her head and the innocent echo of laughter opened me. It was a fleeting second, gone as fast as it came, but it was an ancient echo that I thought I had forgotten. My passage into Moment went unnoticed to her, but not by me.

We went to the next stall. Again, she checked each flower arrangement and bartered a price. This one was satisfactory. We collected the bouquets, hopped on our bikes and weaved our way through the traffic towards the restaurant.

Lying in the background, still ringing, was the rich, familiar tone of her laughter. I had traveled far to hear it again.

The next day Roland and I met for coffee. I said, "Rachel is quite beautiful. I'm really attracted to her."

Roland laughed. "Talk about being attracted to unavailable women!"

I had already shared with Roland my propensity for self-sabotage in relationships. Either I would fall for women I couldn't have, or get close to love and run like hell. Since Lydia died and I entered too quickly another relationship, I had been too emotionally raw to sustain a partnership with another woman. I was not made to be alone, but I didn't know how I could be with someone either. It was torturous to spend my days in perpetual solitaire, and equally excruciating to be with someone, someone that may die, or just leave. It was a chasm yet to be breached.

I said to Roland, "What the hell are you talking about?"

His laughing, far from amusing to begin with, continued. "She runs a meditation center. She's part of a religious group that frowns on relationships. She's like a nun."

"A nun? How long has she been doing it?"

"About eleven years."

"Eleven years!"

My countenance must have dropped a notch or two because Roland's laughter started bordering on hysterical. I never violated another's spiritual path. To honor another's path was to honor mine. I shook my head, "Eleven years. Damn!"

Rachel and I had lunch about a month before I was to leave Thailand. She was on her way to visit India the next week. There was a sense of relief sitting with Rachel. I was truly happy for her. The one thing that kept traveling through my mind was "it's good to see you're okay."

People come into our lives, people leave. I don't know why, or even if there is a why. But sitting with Rachel that afternoon I felt a completeness, like the feeling I had sitting on the edge of Lake Lucerne in Brunnen. It was enough. I needed no more than to know she was okay.

She looked at her watch. Her face changed. She taught English at Chiang Mai University and she was late for a class. She jumped up and said, "I'm sorry. I've got to go." It was reminiscent of Cinderella at the stroke of midnight. She rushed off and left me there, full of peace. The echo remembered me and I remembered the echo.

I returned to Lampang. She went off to India. Before I left Thailand I received a letter from Rachel. Her handwriting flowed just like her spirit. Her words were supportive, friendly.

I read the letter, shook my head and muttered, "Eleven years. Damn."

The Taoist story of the boy and the bell did not end when he rang the bell. He did not die at the convergence of sound and echo. He thought he had come to the end of his life, but sound and echo gave the boy more than memory. It filled him with Moment. He lived way into his hundreds, each morning rising to ring the bell, never again to take Moment for granted.

Rachel opened an echo in me. Three brief encounters — a conversation, a meal and a cup of tea brought me home somehow. But it also brought hunger — pain and hunger — for someone to enter my life and for the gift of entering another's. The yearning to love again expanded and contracted me. The cruelty of echo was the memory of sound.

It reminded me of the time Matt and I sat at the Grand Canyon talking about God and Matt said, "Yeah, if I was Pandora I'd be really pissed." I understood what Matt meant. To love, or to even want to love, opened me to yearning, misery, and the most wondrous beauty life has to offer – to love, or to even want to love.

Too Old to Be Young,
Too Young to Be Old

In New Zealand even the dirt's clean. I stepped off the plane in Auckland to bright blue skies and a harbor filled with sails. The crisp, cool air filled my lungs as I took a deep breath.

I didn't really know what I was doing in New Zealand. It was just a stop off for a month and a half. The writing course in Sydney didn't start till the middle of April and I decided that since this would probably be my only shot at seeing New Zealand, I'd just drop by.

I was drawn to New Zealand, just as I was drawn to Thailand. The interplay of past, present and future had once again drawn me into its gravitational pull. I traveled both islands in New Zealand. I stayed in a town for as long as my wandering allowed, usually a day or two, then hopped back on the bus and went to the next town. I was restless in my wanderings, never able to stay long anywhere.

The south island brought me more face to face with me. There was something in the land beneath me. The feel of the earth in Thailand had been soft, lush and gentle; it seemed to spread over me with an ancient shroud. Here, New Zealand's land mass felt new, as crisp as its air. New Zealand mountain peaks were sharp, imposing. Thailand's mountains rolled melodiously. New Zealand's landscape was a crescendo, powerful in its vitality. The rivers in New Zealand sang of youth, tickling rocks still in infancy. The lakes had a youthful playfulness whereas Thailand's lakes and rivers moseyed with age and their smile was more a smile of well-earned wisdom.

New Zealand was everything I wasn't. I had aged, weathered by loss. I felt old in soul and body. It had been two years since Matt's death.

There are so many positive aspects I have found in the Afterloss, but the physical and emotional depletion was overwhelming. I would wake in the morning and it was there with me. I'd walk the coastlines and it walked me. No matter where I went, what I did, the depletion left me perpetually low, and my fear was that this exhaustion would never leave.

I was witness to New Zealand's beauty, bounding energy and vitality. It measured me in contrast and I saw an old man, slipping away, slipping back into a point of reference of what had been, defined by what was. It was not pleasant to sit by the waters of New Zealand and feel their flow. The reflection it showed me made me feel as if I'd gone gray overnight. Grief had lost movement again and the sheer strength of New Zealand, her majestic beauty coupled with her youthful spirit, sent me further asunder.

I fell into a cavernous past, ominously dark. My energy supplies had run out.

I couldn't break free. In a desperate attempt to move forward I had fallen hopelessly backwards.

The echo of the tower bell in the folktale, the rich resonance of heartbeat I felt in Rachel's laugh, had followed me to New Zealand. She had come and gone in my life. She was okay and that was enough. We shared Moment, sound and echo, and it was over. But just as New Zealand mirrored my aging, Rachel's laugh was a reflection of all that I no longer possessed, or thought possible to possess again.

Kaikoura sits on the western shores of the south island. The small town attracts a lot of tourists with its beauty and the opportunity to swim with the dolphins. I decided to go to the dolphins rather than wait for them to come to me in Monterey.

A group of passing strangers sat in the small backroom of the dive shop. We were instructed in the art of dolphin attraction. A dolphin would only approach out of curiosity. So, we were told to make the most bizarre noises through our snorkels and most likely a dolphin would come to see what it was. They warned us that these dolphins were wild and were not to be touched. It wasn't a rerun of Flipper.

In our thick wetsuits, goggles, masks, fins and snorkels we were carted out to sea. The guide searched the water's surface for dolphin pods. My fellow travelers wanted to swim with dolphins, but I was there wanting more. I wanted to know why no dolphin jumped that day in Monterey.

When I hit the frigid waters I made a bizarre noise all right. I acclimated to the waters and went in search for dolphins. All around the boat high pitched sounds blared through the snorkels. There was a sense of gaiety and lightness in the others. The dolphins began to gather, dip close to someone and then dive to the depths. Occasionally people would raise their heads out of the water and laugh. I was not laughing.

A dolphin came near to me, but at a safe distance. I made a noise somewhere between a cry and a squeal. Her eyes scanned my hand, and then looked into my mask. I was just another anomaly that had entered her world. Only seconds passed before she tore off into the blue, gliding effortlessly out of my sight.

God, how I wanted to touch her before she left. How I wanted one of these glorious creatures to stop for more than just a few seconds. To answer me.

Only a mask separated the salt of my tears from the salt of an ocean.

Once again, my present tense was ruled by my past. While the other tourists had fun, I was still drenched with cold wind and rain at an aquarium in Monterey, still waiting for dolphins to jump, or at the very least to understand why they didn't. I was still looking for something in this world to explain the world just beyond my reach.

Deep in the eastern part of New Zealand's south island, many kilometers from Kaikoura, I sat by a river. Crystal clear mountain streams swept to the sea. What I wouldn't have given to have a rose in hand, but there were no death days, no birthdays to rest my sorrow. I was alone with me.

The river and I sat next to each other, her in her movement, and me in stagnation. I tossed pebbles into her and they disappeared in the way a thought disappears into the void. Rose petals float. Pebbles sink.

Was loss the measure of me?

The river held me briefly in my own reflection. I was still weary, still trying to crawl out of a dream of five relics in a wooden box, still counting days between roses, still looking for three dolphins to jump in an ocean, still hearing the faint echo of a bell tower. I was still collecting a past more than a present, still sitting by rivers tossing pebbles, still alone.

I said a little prayer. "God, either give me a life or take this one. I've had enough."

Some Corners Aren't Corners At All

I flew into Sydney at night, weary more in soul than body. The experiences in Thailand and New Zealand had taken an inner toll. I wasn't sure I was going to be able to turn the corner.

Turning the corner was a concept I used to lean heavily on, as if there was a corner to turn. In my relationship with loss I kept the sense that somewhere, somehow, this was going to change. My mantra for many years was "this too shall pass." I would wait the night to wait the day, waiting for that magical corner to appear.

The corner that I so desperately wanted to turn was intrinsically connected to time. If I were told that this pain and sorrow would end in nine years, seven months, three weeks and two days, I'd say okay. I could make it nine years, seven months, three weeks and two days. My only question would be "Will that be in the am or pm?" Ironically, it was timelessness I feared the most.

I had to make peace with time in order to move beyond what was.

Roland helped me settle in. A friend of his was selling a flat in Darlinghurst, just across the road from King's Cross.

It felt good to have a place to stay longer than two nights in a row. Finally I had a place to unpack and settle in for a while.

The writing course started three days later. Maybe the corner was there.

The class had about twelve people, plus Roland. The last student was late, fifteen minutes to be exact.

Ioana was good at making an entrance. Her long brown hair was set as meticulously as her tan pants, color coordinated sports coat and silk scarf. She looked to the left of the circle of desks, looked to the right, and then settled into the one directly across from me.

I captivate easily. And it was easy to be captivated by Ioana. She had an urban air of poise. Her words clipped with confidence. Her brown eyes collected quickly anything that moved. Ioana was both poetry and power in motion. She was Romanian by birth. Her family escaped Communist rule by fleeing with nothing when she was fourteen. They left a middle class world of Romania for a shared shelter in Germany, ultimately to find their way to Australia. She spoke several languages, had graduated with top marks and secured a professional position in the corporate world with ease.

She was determined, driven by some destinational force. Ioana kept her eye on the prize and she seemed quite clear on the list of prizes she had in mind.

She enrolled in the writing course to re-energize a movie script she had begun. She had read extensively on the subject of screenplays, their structure and commercial potentiality. Ioana was not one to leave anything to chance.

I fell in love with Ioana. She saved my life. And it damn near killed me in the process.If any relationship entailed "the agony and the ecstasy," it was the year-long relationship I had with Ioana. She brought me back to the living. Her love and care was as strong as her inner being.

I gleaned a great deal from her. She seemed to have an infinite reserve and the ability to put it to practice. Ioana pulled me out of time's darkness. But at the same time, the relationship reminded me of electrical cardiac arrest pads. Powerful surges of energy jerked me back into life, but boy, it sure hurts.

Ioana and I broke up, got together and broke up again. Our common ground, beginning with creativity and all the pleasures that brings, began to fade, and inevitably, so did we. We did our best to move in the same direction, but we both gave up too much of ourselves to have enough left to build a life together. Ioana had the good sense to call it quits. And I had the good sense to agree.

But she gave me a gift – a beating heart, and a place for it to beat. I sincerely thought this was the corner that I was to turn. For a brief moment it felt like I had escaped the gravitational pull of my past and the present tasted of pleasure, excitement and hope.

Who the hell said hope springs eternal?

Even though we agreed to go our separate ways, and it was truly for the best, it was difficult to see that corner fade right before my eyes.

I was not born to do life alone. The chasm between the heart's desire and the state of the heart was too great. And there seemed to be no bridge between the two. I was trapped in two worlds – the one that said I want to share my life with someone and the other world that said I do not have the capacity to lose one more person.

The loss of a dream with Ioana brought to the surface the loss of all my dreams. Loss did not discriminate between another failed relationship and the death of Bryan, Lydia and Matt. Nothing resides in isolation, especially loss.

However, the other side of loss's inability to compartmentalize was that it would not let me surrender my capacity to love. If I was to embrace loss, I had to embrace love as well.

I thought loss was a journey into sorrow. I didn't realize until I ventured to its depths that it was a journey into love, too.

The embers that were lit with Rachel's laugh in Chiang Mai spread across me with Ioana's gift. If I could live through other losses, I could live through this loss. And equally important, if I could love once, then I could love again. Sometimes to find a corner, I have to back track a little.

The River Bends

"I think we should follow the river," Rachel said.

I rested against a fallen tree to catch my breath. "Okay."

It had been three hours of walking, two and half-hours lost in Doi Inthanon, a large national park in Thailand. We had no water or food. We thought the cryptic map we got from the guesthouse was enough to have a nice stroll up a portion of the mountain. We thought the hot Thailand sun would send us back to the guesthouse in about an hour. But in the thick foliage we became completely disoriented. The trail disappeared, just like us.

No one knew we were out there except the elderly lady at the guesthouse. And we had no illusions that the Thai government was going to put out an all points bulletin on two farangs (foreigners) in the jungle, at least not for a day or two.

Thick bush and fallen trees blocked the river every hundred yards or so. We had to climb the ravine on more than one occasion, keeping close to the river as possible. It was our only hope. Water would lead us to civilization.

Our steps depleted us, but the afternoon sun's steady pace into night and our heightening concern kept us moving.

This walk in the middle of a Thai jungle was a far cry from our first walk in Sydney, Australia just three months earlier. I was living alone in Bondi, an eastern suburb of Sydney. Rachel still lived in Thailand, but she flew into Australia to lead some seminars for her spiritual organization.

It had been over a year and a half since I saw Rachel at our lunch in Chiang Mai. We did not have any contact for seven or eight months. However, Roland was in the process of starting an online writing group through The Writer's Studio. He asked for volunteers to participate in the pilot project. I agreed. So did Rachel.

Our writing over the net deepened our friendship. One of the exercises Roland asked the group to do was take a word and write. Rachel and I took this practice a little further. We agreed to exchange words, one at a time. The exercise had three rules. One was to write immediately upon opening the email. The second was to write whatever came in that stream of consciousness. And three, send it back without editing any part.

Christians have a scripture verse about Jesus that says, "The word became flesh." In our writing I also saw how flesh becomes word.

The power of a word unfolds the wordsmith. I put aside the editor within and the critic. And when I opened to the word it opened me. I was as much surprised as anyone where one word can go, its height and width, the flow of direction turning, pirouetting and in the twinkling of an eye turning again, sometimes in on itself, sometimes heading out into the expanse, sometimes fading into the infinite. And now I was sending stream of conscious writing to Rachel, unedited, unprotected.

Rachel touches life gently. Her smooth caress of my words was healing. Her words, unedited, unprotected, were equally healing. It was a sacred exchange of layers unshared in a lifetime, but familiar in their touch. Each morning I was given the gift of building a trust in someone that I had this instinctive desire to trust.

Rachel had the capacity to enter the enclosure within me and draw me out into the open. We slowly inched our way there, word by word.

Oddly enough, as I waited for Rachel at the airport in Sydney I didn't remember what she looked liked. I remembered her blonde hair. The ocean blue of her eyes was more in the memory of the heart than the memory of the mind. What lodged in my heart was the memory of her spirit.

As soon as Rachel started her descent down the ramp the heart and mind met. Like the old Taoist monk that heard the bell again after so many years away, this time Rachel's smile on that ramp resonated memory.

Words on a page segued easily into conversation. We spoke from mid-sentence, and we spoke into the night.

But before night there was our first walk. We walked the famous coastal trek from Bondi to Bronte in Sydney. The concrete path curved the cliffs. The ocean beneath us pushed against rock edges and the boulders that broke away centuries ago. On the way to Bronte she said she was in transition. She had decided to explore another way of life. She was leaving the group to which she had dedicated her life to for twelve years. It was a big move and Rachel moves slowly into major decisions. And nothing could be more major than the shifting of a belief system.

My journey from West to East had not been easy. I shared with her my experience of standing on my own precipice. We strolled through the sacredness of Spirit as our steps slowly moved on the footpath.

On the way to Bronte we shared a deep friendship. On our return walk to Bondi we shared a deep silence. In the hour walk from Bronte to Bondi neither one of us spoke. We walked without a need to voice ourselves, as if to speak would diminish us. When my fingers curled into hers she looked into my eyes with a slight smile.

The silence shaped us that day.

We returned to Bondi. I guided us off the concrete path onto the long stretch of beach. Winter had driven the bathers indoors and we sat pretty much in seclusion in the sand, almost eye level to the smooth Pacific.

A kiss sealed our silence. Word by word we had found silence, and in silence we had found a kiss.

Months later we were back in Thailand, relieved we at least found a river. We were both calm, but as minutes turned to hours the true extent of our situation was becoming increasingly clear. It would be dark soon. The lack of food and water was compounded by our lack of matches, bedrolls, and most importantly, direction. But we had a river.

Rachel is the epitome of ease coupled with a firm determination. In Chinese astrology I'm a fire monkey. Rachel is a water tiger. Water tiger describes her well. There is a reservoir of quiet strength within her that is relentless.

She put one foot in front of another on the soft riverbank without complaint. She did what needed to be done. If we had to scale the side of cliff, she scaled it. If we were knee deep in the rushing water, her steps were steady. Leeches were dislodged as if she was just readjusting a bracelet. Her strength travels in softness; her softness traveled in me.

On most of the trek Rachel took the lead. I guess it was because Thailand was her turf. I just assumed she knew what she was doing. I thought she'd taken these kinds of treks many times in her seven years in Chiang Mai. It was an erroneous assumption. It would be likened to her following me lost in Yosemite just because I lived in California, but I liked watching her walk anyway.

We stopped to rest. There were leaves in her disheveled hair and mud on her face and clothes. She was as beautiful as I had ever seen her, simply radiant. She wasn't even looking at me when Moment appeared. She was looking down the river, judging our steps to the next detour over another fallen tree that blocked our watercourse way. I felt absolutely at home, within myself, within her, within Moment. She turned back to me, my eyes still encircling her. She smiled and said, "Ready?"

I smiled. "Yeah, I'm ready."

I had no doubt we would make it. I didn't know how, or when, but walking down the mountain, following the river, I knew. No harm could possibly come to such a beautiful creature. And I was with her.

Thirty minutes more downstream we saw a blue irrigation pipe, our first signs of civilization in over four hours. It was only one section of plastic discarded by the overgrown creek. It gave us no clue to the distance left. Daylight still filtered through the trees, but the angle of shadow warned us that we didn't have long. Still, we neither hurried nor slowed. We just kept going.

The river led to a road. We emerged from the jungle muddy, tired and with scratches all over our arms and necks. A small band of Thai soldiers lounged at a guard post. Their surprise turned to laughter when they saw two farangs stumble onto the road. Rachel said something in Thai and they pointed down the road.

I was grateful to get back to the guesthouse around dusk. We showered the day off our skin. It felt good to be clean and fed. We laid our bodies down early that night. She was about to fall asleep in my arms. I thought back over the day. Maybe, just maybe, I'm ready.

Thirty Minutes from Here

Rachel had been doing volunteer work with the Karen refugees in Northern Thailand for over three years. The project was to assist children of war through teacher training programs. The educational material focused on helping children come to terms with war through avenues of peace. Lesson plans, songs and games took the child from the fear, anger, hate and loss, through the living pain to living peace. It offered a direction out of the cycle of sorrow through a process of relearning what it is like to play, to laugh, to be safe, to be a child. Rachel ventured several times a year to the northern border between Thailand and Myanmar to train the teachers.

For centuries the Karen have been fierce warriors, a proud people. But after the uprising in 1988 when the military took over Burma and renamed their country Myanmar, the Karen have been a hunted people. There are many refugee camps scattered across the northwest of Thailand, just beyond the reach of the military junta of Myanmar, and just beyond the reach of their home.

Rachel and I rode in the back of a covered pickup truck with the supplies for the six-hour ride up to Mae Hong Son. We rested on boxes of pens, paper, some soccer balls, and sweets, precious gifts to a people with little. Another two-hour trek up the dirt mountain roads to the village awaited us.

When we passed the Thai security and inched our way to the heart of Section One I was surprised at the idyllic view of the green plush vegetation climbing the side of the mountain. The tips of teak-leaf roofs nestled serenely in the trees. A Hilton Hotel couldn't have found a more picturesque view. It was a beautiful land, but it was Thailand, not their Burma, now Myanmar. A forced encampment, no matter what it looks like on the outside, was still a prison surrounded by guards. A paradise with borders is no paradise at all.

Peter, the camp leader, met us. He was a thoughtful man short in height. His dark black hair was thick; his eyes coal black. Peter was a school principal back home. He welcomed the help, the supplies and the opportunity to speak to us. We sat on the floor in his home that consisted of bamboo walls set on stilts. He spoke of the trials and tribulations of living in the refugee camp. He daily juggled the needs of the Thai authorities and the people under his care. He was the focal point of three worlds – Thailand, the camp, and a world that still lives in the refugee.

The camp was like any community forced to make do far from home. There were people of great beauty, radiant in spirit, open and giving. There were also the greedy ones with dull eyes and bloated fingers red from holding too tightly whatever they could. There were the ones that walked weary on the dirt paths carrying the weight of memory. And still others that had the fragrance of gratitude for a place of peace, regardless of how transitory it was. There were the ones filled with hope living alongside the hopeless.

One old man we walked past sat in his house staring down the path. His thin hand wiped his forehead slowly down across his cheek to his chin. He looked from the distance at the strangers. He turned from us, disinterested, as if to say it doesn't matter why you are here, nothing matters. He had no anger, no fear, no joy, no-thing. He was drained of purpose in this paradise.

I turned away. I didn't want to lessen the proud man anymore than I already had just by walking by his house in a land not his home.

The most telling feature of life in the refugee camp was time. The day held too much time. The years held too little. But the camp held another time, thirty minutes to be exact. This community of one hundred thousand, just a small fraction compared to the population of thirty-five million still in Myanmar, kept time by their country's watch, which is thirty minutes behind.

I understood that kind of timekeeping. Time kept memory alive, time kept hope close, but time enclosed and bound both, just as the loss that measured my time did.

In these beautiful surroundings there was layer upon layer of loss that hung on the morning mist, invisible in the daylight and covered by the night air. It took me a few days to see the similarities between their way of keeping time and mine. It took longer to realize we were both grieving.

I still kept time with loss's time. I was in love with Rachel. Her ease and adaptability to any situation anywhere rested me closer to real time, but I still could not breach the distance. There was always something that would draw me back into loss's time.

Children are a pure reflection of a community. They have yet to find the masks that hide a wide-open heart. Mrs. Hammert, Matt's kindergarten teacher, once said that she knew more about the families of her children than anybody on the planet. The kids held the family secrets and didn't know the secrets were to be held.

The eyes of the Karen children and their smiling laughter held the community's sorrow. They may not have known the uncle that was murdered in front of their mother, or the grandparent the father can only speak of in past tense because the soldiers came through in the night.

In fact, many of the children were born in the camp, homeless at birth. But still they carried this pervading mist of loss behind rich chocolate eyes, and it echoed in their radiant laughter.

There is a tonal quality to laughter born of sorrow. These children had color to their laugh, and the expanse of a universe in the color of night in those brown eyes.

The Karen children's eyes were Matt's eyes. Their laugh echoed Matt's. But even more telling, each person I encountered was a reflection of me. The good and the bad were me. The ones living in scarcity, the ones that gave unconditionally, the greedy ones, the empty ones, the hopeless and the hopeful all reflected a part of me. Their stories were my stories. They may have different external languages and landscapes, but the interior of them was the interior of me.

The teachers gathered in the common area. Not surprisingly, we started about thirty minutes late. Rachel led the meeting. She held the teachers with openness and a loving spirit. In Thailand there is a phrase for people like Rachel. It's jai yin. It means a kind heart. Rachel guided the meeting with a kind heart.

The teachers told of their successes in teaching the children the material and how it was making a difference. Children of war take war into their lives, into the classroom and into adulthood. Opening a way of peace in the class was an opening into another way to deal with conflict. The teachers shared how arguments were settled peacefully, reconciliation happened by using the principles taught in the curriculum. The teachers were happy that their jobs were made easier.

We joined a class in action. Edward, the teacher, was in his early thirties, but his youthful exuberance made him look around eighteen. His bright white smile was infectious. His loose curly black locks of hair stopped just at the edge of his neck. He had the eyes of a child in wonder and his laugh was the same color of the children that clearly adored him. Edward was in his element. He was born for the stage. The electricity of his movements kept the children spell bound.

Later that night, in his bamboo house, Edward showed me where the bullet lodged in his chest during the 1988 protest and consequent uprising in Rangoon. He told the story of how he was rushed out of the darkness into hiding. His body healed enough to make it out of the city.

His soul was still healing. He was a teacher now. He taught the children about forgiveness, the most powerful weapon of war. But it was clear that Edward still lived thirty minutes away from where we sat that night.

Time and distance. When Jim said in Mendocino that my grief would take time and distance to heal, I thought I knew time. I thought I knew distance. But until I tried to wed the two, I didn't know the extent of the two.

The Karen taught me just how loss bends time to her own accord. It was there in their isolation that I found mine being mirrored. They were safe, in beauty, the food was lacking abundance, but there was enough. They had roofs over their heads. They had everything but time. Instead, time had them as it had me.

This aberration of time kept the days and years at bay. It was survival that dictated a day lived out of sync with the land beneath them. It was not defiance that kept them in Karen time. It was hope that someday they would get to go home.

And the years? The years that had passed in the camp became bearable as long as they were thirty minutes different. The year ahead could be endured if it was filtered through the hourglass thirty minutes away. And it was not just the passing years, but the fading years as well that somehow became possible to bear.

I lay next to Rachel under the same cloud of time. We pushed our thin mats on the small hut floor closer together. The one-hour of electricity allotted in the night had long since passed and the other huts that dotted the mountain were quiet and still. The candle illumined her as she lay in her sleeping bag next to me; and I was caught in Time's between. I wanted to hold her in real time, but something kept me thirty minutes away.

If I let go of loss's time, what would be left of me? Would the past fade? Would the change in time bring more pain, more than I could absorb? In other relationships this was as far as I could go. Love had this innate border crossing that I was unable to enter. But Rachel held a unique space. I was drawn to her love by the way she loved as much as by her capacity to love. She neither pushed nor pulled. She simply was, which made it simple to be.

The relationship between love and loss was tangled in time. The more I loved the more I lost. The more I studied the chasm between my ability to love and the enormous barrier of my fear of loss I saw just how trapped I was.

Rachel and I walked the winding footpaths in the camp from section to section, up the mountain passes, balancing on loose rocks to cross the river. We rested often while our guides waited for us to catch our breaths. They had learned to breathe in the enclosed space. It was nothing for them to carry great weights on these narrow paths. They once roamed their homeland balancing on precipices far more challenging than the tame land they could not leave. Our guides waited as long as we needed.

I followed Rachel into the Karen refugee camp. When we left to return to Chiang Mai I was to follow the inner workings of time, its causes and consequences. I was falling deeper in love, which meant I was falling further into loss.

Time and distance. Pain and pleasure. Love and loss.

Somewhere, somehow, if I could only find peace with time I might find where time and timelessness meet. The price of loving again was to follow whatever came emotionally, physically, mentally and spiritually. To not close down, but to follow loss, hopefully to the end of time.

With This Ring

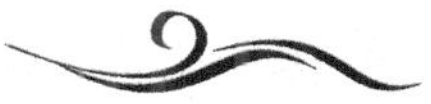

Rachel and I settled briefly in Chiang Mai. We knew we were heading back to Australia in about three months.

One way Rachel made ends meet was to write travel and feature articles for newspapers and in-flight magazines. It didn't cost a lot to live in Thailand, but wages were low as well. If she could sell an article, she would be set for a month or two.

She wanted to do an article on the Buddhist temples in Luang Praban in Laos. We climbed aboard a night bus to Chiang Rai and then another bus took us to the border of Thailand and Laos along the Mei Kong River.

Once we crossed the Mei Kong River into Laos we asked about the best way to get to Luang Praban. We had a mutual travel philosophy – why plan ahead? Whatever comes, go with it. It was easy to travel with Rachel.

We had three choices. One was to fly. By western standards it was a fairly cheap, but we were living close to the bone, saving where we could for our return to Australia. The second was a boat with no sleeping quarters that took three days and we had heard through the proverbial grapevine of backpackers it was pretty grueling. The last alternative was a jet boat. It took eight hours. The jet engine would be tied to the back of a long thin boat with wooden benches, two to a row. And we would soar inches above the river's surface at breakneck speed.

We sat at the travel agent's office in the border town. I looked at Rachel. I said, "We've just spent all night riding a bus with no sleep. Let's fly, at least up there."

Laos was beautiful from the air. The dark green landscape felt rich and ancient. Rivers carved by nature's time meandered with aged sacredness within the jungles. Even the hum of the engines couldn't drown the silence of the forests below us.

Our budget did not allow for a plane trip back. We were forced to choose between the jet boat and the three-day endurance test on the slow ship. We chose the jet boat. For eight long, long hours we sat with our elbows in our armpits, teeth chattering, and brain jarring speed, just inches from the murky waters. The only diversion from my thoughts of being flung out onto the shallow rocks just beneath the surface was the intermittent pouring rain that pelted our faces like stinging needles. We made it across the border to Thailand just before the customs office closed. I slept with the sound of a jet engine still rattling in my head, but grateful for the nice guesthouse bed and the mosquito net.

People my age usually have careers, homes, cars, retirement plans, kids, and grandchildren on the horizon. Before I passed out from exhaustion, I thought, "What the hell am I doing here?" Our bodies curved each others, enclaved by the mattress. The smell of Rachel's freshly washed hair filled me and in my next breath came the next question, "How did I get so blessed?"

The Most Out of Each Day

Our next adventure sent us south. Roland was taking another group of writers to Thailand. This time it was down to Phi Phi Island. Rachel could take the course for free if she coordinated the arrangements. So, we took the overnight train from Chiang Mai to Bangkok, a bus from Bangkok to Krabi, and from Krabi a boat to Phi Phi Island. To top off this escapade of buses, boats and trains we had decided to do a seven-day cleansing fast. No food for seven days. Foolishly we started the fast the day before we left Chiang Mai.

The second day of any fast is usually the hardest. Unfortunately, we had to spend six hours in the Bangkok train station waiting for our connection. Even more unfortunate was that the only place there was air-conditioning was in the cafeteria. It was a test of endurance, but we were in it together. Hour after hour we blessed the breeze of the air-conditioning on empty stomachs. Moment by moment Rachel and I were building shared history.

Phi Phi Island was beautiful. Pristine waters surrounded the lush land. Smaller islands dotted the horizon in the near distance. The streets were just wide enough for walking and the beaches spread with white sand curled the coves.

The writers that were to arrive in a couple of days were already booked at an upscale hotel. Rachel made sure everything was ready and waiting for them so we went off looking for where we would stay. We looked for something a bit more modest. But as we walked the main town with backpacks in tow we discovered that the guesthouses did not have middle of the road rooms. Either they were little holes with walls or nice lovely rooms a bit on the pricey side. We had pretty much hit all of the "hole with walls" as night approached. At the end of town was a hotel landscaped on the side of the small mountain. Individual cottages were nestled in palm trees. I said to Rachel, "Let's go check it out."

She looked at me with a soft, sympathetic smile like a mother would look at her child when he announces, "I'm going to be an astronaut when I grow up."

I said, "Well, at least we can go look at a room."

Compared to what we'd seen, the room was wonderful. The view was stunning. I looked at Rachel with my best puppy dog eyes.

I had two objectives on our trip to Phi Phi. The first was to write a play. While Rachel took her class I was going to write this play that had been rattling around my head for a while. The second objective, much more important than the first, was to share a commitment ceremony with Rachel. We had talked about doing a ring exchange and a little ceremony to externally voice our desire to journey together.

I wanted the place we stayed to be conducive to both. We left the hotel and sat on the beach. We discussed the pros and cons of all the places we'd looked at that day. My vote was on the last one.

By U.S. standards this lovely Phi Phi island hotel was about the price of a Motel 6, but by our standards it was high. The money I started with after Matt died was still dwindling. It was running more on the side of empty than full. The days with Rachel were slowly shifting me.

For many years, the staying alive as long as the money lasted was what kept me alive. There was some internal pact I made with myself that no matter the degree of darkness I traveled I would not finish this life until all my resources had run dry. Ironically, it kept death at bay. I had hoped that if I just stayed alive long enough I would find a reason to live beyond just the observation of loss. I had two futures in wait. One was death by poverty. The other was life by meaning, and I believed meaning would bring the flow of money.

On the beach at Phi Phi Island, I wanted a life of meaning.

Rachel was not the source of my love; Rachel was the recipient of my love. I used to get the two confused with other women, which ultimately led to the inevitable downfall of my relationships. I would start looking for a finite being to provide what only the Infinite could. Nothing transitory can truly sustain a spirit. And I know of only one source that isn't transitory.

My writing wasn't my meaning either. Writing grounds me, paints me, colors me in time and space, but it, too, was a recipient of meaning, not the source.

On the beach I said to Rachel, "It's more than just the money. It's a statement to the Universe that we're worth it. I want to write and I can write there. I don't want to be typing away in the corner of a dark, pokey room with a cheap fan. Been there, done that. I want sunlight. Air-conditioning. This will be a real statement. Besides, let's look at this as our honeymoon. I want us to do our ceremony from that balcony that looks out over the ocean. We'll be all right. I truly believe that if you do what you love, the Universe shows up with the cash. I don't know how, but I know it does."

It was a beautiful day on that balcony. April 1ˢᵗ, 2000. April Fool's Day. We had gathered elements of the land, air and sea. A feather, some sand, salt water and other gifts of the earth decorated the hotel tray that sat between us. The day before we had found a street vendor selling rings for about one U.S. dollar. We splurged and bought two. The words we shared were gifted solely for the other. I slid the ring on her finger; the matching ring eased on my left hand. Instead of cutting a cake we split open a Kit Kat. Then we took the elements of the earth down to the sea. It was high tide when we spoke our final vows and lowered the tray into the gentle lapping wave.

No dramatic statements or ornate gestures marked this outward display of our commitment. It was as gentle and natural as Rachel herself. It mirrored her true nature as her moments do. I was struck by the serenity that surrounded me in my opening to her.

But it took great effort for me to create the space within me for such a moment. Rings and commitment scared me. Not just because they mean forever, but also because I know just how transient forever is. Before the ceremony I could tell I was starting to internally distance from Rachel. I shared with her how the rings and their meaning of forever frightened me and how I was starting to distance.

She said, "Yeah, forever frightens me, too. Why don't we look at the rings as being a symbol of getting the most out of each day? It doesn't have to mean forever."

My distance dissolved.

Ironically, the cheap rings lasted just a few days before they broke. We laughed and tossed them in the ocean, too. It was a year later before we did another ring exchange on the edge of another ocean in another land. And a ring didn't have to mean forever. A ring could mean to make the most out of every day. A ring could be a symbol of Moment itself. What I learned from Matt I was now beginning to live within me with Rachel.

The Richest Man on Earth

Rachel and I needed to apply for visas in order to get back into Australia. She returned to England every year to see her family and it seemed logical that we would apply there. It just so happened that my father had a business meeting in London around the same time we were planning to go to see her father and brothers, sister-in-laws and eight nephews. My mother rarely traveled, but the prospect of meeting Rachel enticed her to join the rendezvous in London. This would be the first time I was to meet Rachel's clan and the first time for Rachel to meet my folks, coupled with the introductions of the two families.

We landed at Heathrow Airport a week before my parent's arrival. Her father, John, met us there and drove us down to Mangotsfield, a quiet little suburb of Bristol. John's sweet spirit was glowing when he caught sight of Rachel. John lived alone in the same house that Rachel had grown up in. Over forty years of memory lingered in the old Victorian home.

The feel of Rachel's mother, Jean, was strong. She painted as a hobby and her artwork hung on the walls of the stairs. The stairway still had the chair lift she used to get from the bedroom down to the rest of the house.

Before our journey Rachel and I shared long conversations of how loss molds to the moment in a unique way. I had yet to lose a parent. She had never had children, much less had one die. To lose a parent seemed to me to be a rite of passage, a natural progression with a particular weight and length. She could give to me an understanding I had yet to experience. I, on the other hand, shared the uniqueness of a child's death. The beauty of our interchange was that the individual circumstances of death that were foreign to the other found common ground in Spirit.

The touch of the banister and Jean's paintings drew me more than any other room. But it was in John that I was able to see Jean best. No one who loves lives in isolation and there is a distinct hue that permeates a soul that has loved.

Rachel's love added a unique color to my capacity to love. Experiencing her family helped me round out my understanding of her and the journey she traveled.

Rachel and I took a bus from Bristol to London. My folks' hotel was close to downtown, but we stayed with Rachel's Aunt Didi.

Didi's journey included schizophrenia. Whereas my brother Michael's schizophrenia had left him unable to work or function easily in the world around him, Didi was able to hold a job for many years, ultimately retiring.

Didi was gentle in spirit, in voice and manner. There was a special place for Didi in Rachel. Didi was rather quiet, her spirit didn't take up much room, but the space in which her spirit spread had a healing silhouette.

Didi reminded me of the children's story of the Velveteen Rabbit. The story is about a stuffed rabbit that is loved so much that she loses her buttons and her fur; she becomes frayed and old, but the love gave life to the toy and the rabbit became real. Didi was not frayed. Her gray hair was meticulously kept. Her make-up was in subtle proportions and well placed. She carried herself with dignity and grace, but the realness that rested upon her was through the years of pain and sorrow, and her ability to love. Her fraying was of an internal nature. The winds of life had created a beauty in Didi, a beauty born and lived in realness.

Besides the meeting of families, the task Rachel and I had was to go to the Australian embassy in London and secure our visas. We waited with applications in hand at the bus stop for the double decker that would take us downtown. Ten minutes passed, and a number of buses, just not ours. Twenty minutes passed, still no number with our destination. Thirty minutes.

Around forty minutes into the wait I said to Rachel, "You know you're rich when you can get into a taxi and not care how much it costs."

The bus finally arrived. We made it to the Embassy, took a ticket and waited some more. The kind lady at the counter took our applications. Then she informed us that we needed medical exams. We needed a chest X-ray and some other tests.

We found a doctor, but we could not make our appointments for the same day. Rachel went first. While Rachel was at the doctor Didi and I went window shopping. We returned to the waiting room to wait. Rachel was told that she had to have another check-up at a special breast clinic. Calmly she said, "They found three lumps on my breast. They have to do a biopsy and a scan."

Her voice was matter of fact and carried no sense of danger. My thoughts didn't match her voice.

She continued, "The only time they can fit me in is in forty-five minutes."

She told us the location. Didi said, "There isn't time to get there by bus or the Tube. We're going to have to take a taxi."

The black old-fashioned taxi was spacious. Didi and Rachel sat facing the front. I was in the seat that faced them, but I couldn't face them. I was fighting the tears with very little success. If I looked at Rachel I would have been completely undone.

It was embarrassing, but I couldn't help it. Didi was calm. She wore her thoughts in silence. Rachel wasn't worried in the least. Whatever happened, Rachel could cope. As for me, I was not coping well at all.

I was nowhere near being in that taxi. I was strung together with the memory of another test when Lydia and I sat in her doctor's office, when the needle drew blood and we asked questions of what does it mean if we have HIV, what about the children? My present descended into looking at Lydia at the stoplight, she with Bryan, me with Matt, and that haunting look of helplessness. Then memory stretched through the years, months, days, nights of watching them slowly die. Everything I had passed, passed again. I looked out the window, covering my face as best I could, and fought back the tears.

I realized we were in a taxi. I remembered the bus stop. I looked at Rachel and said, "Do you remember when I said 'you know you're a rich man when you can take a taxi and not care how much it costs?'"

She nodded.

I said, "I'm the richest man alive. Because I don't care how much this taxi costs."

Rachel softly smiled. She touched my leg and said, "It's going to be all right."

She was comforting me. But she could not see a future of what I had seen in the past. The phrase, innocence is bliss, is so true. I thought of what her body would travel through, the mornings, the nights, the pain, the day in and day out slipping away, the parallel universes that would separate us while we lay next to each other, the ethereal conversations that I would try to encase in my memory like trying to cling to mist, and the last breath, the very last breath left that ultimately leaves all else behind, distant and desolate.

Didi and I sat in the waiting room for two hours. My mind was in a cloud of chaos trying its best to dislodge the past from the present. I sat. I paced. I sat again.

Didi watched me without the need for words. She held me with the expanse of her gentle soul. I had only known her for a few days, but the depth of her spirit was familiar to the touch.

I would glance at her and try to smile. The attentiveness of her eyes grounded me.

The tests were finished. Rachel came out with a sheet of paper. She immediately said, "We will know in three days."

We decided not to tell my parents. They had met Rachel and instantly were drawn to her. We didn't want to unduly alarm them. They had been through enough.

Rachel returned to Bristol the next day as planned. I had to wait for my tests so I stayed in London at Didi's longer.

I spent the days with my parents when they were free, with Didi for a few hours here and there and with my footsteps in between. My stillness had more room when I walked. I did a lot of walking.

Didi and I went to the park down the street from her flat. The calmness of her spirit held me as we sat in the coffee shop. This was part of her weekly routine. She'd have a sweet and then proceed to the park bench for a little time feeding the birds and squirrels.

We didn't talk about Rachel on the walk to the park or at the coffee shop. It was just small talk compare to the large talk that was swirling around my brain.

As we were about to leave the coffee shop she stopped to chat to a man with MS in a wheel chair. He smiled at Didi as she approached him. She shared a brief conversation. I did not hear the words as I was just rising from the table, but when I glanced upon the scene of Didi standing next to the man I was struck by the totality of her attention and the touch of her hand on his shoulder. She was so soft and present.

We went out on a stroll around the park. If there is one thing the Brits can do, they can sure put together a beautiful garden. The park was aged like a fine wine. She showed me all the out of the way places where light plays with shadows, flowers glow and the underbrush teems with life. She listened to the birds and I became aware of their melodic conversations. When we sat with bread in hand and birds at our feet, I became aware of being in the present tense because Didi drew me there.

Didi used words sparingly. She could hold long periods of silence comfortably. I always felt her silence was like the soft swaying of long graceful branches in a gentle breeze. When she did speak it was rich.

Out of the context of that moment between idle conversation and silence, Didi said, "She's going to be okay."

I was struck by the unique quality of Didi's presence in the words more than the words themselves. I wasn't even sure the words were going to be true. But it was another time the temporal found its way to eternal.

She slid back into idle conversation leaving me with the aftertaste of tenderness. I did not press her or pursue her. It had passed. She let me glimpse something in her and I honored the privilege by nodding silently in return.

The Shadow of a Footprint

As I paced the streets of London each step stepped into the ones I took years before – the waiting for test results, the scenarios that might unfold, and the dark places that take me under.

Chuang Tzu wrote a parable called *Flight from the Shadow*. It is about a man that was so upset at the sight of his shadow and disturbed by his own footsteps that he tried to rid himself of both. He decided the only way to do this was to run away. But every step created another footprint and no matter how fast he ran the shadow kept pace. The man thought that if he only ran faster then he would be able to escape. So, he ran so hard and for so long that he dropped dead from exhaustion. Chuang Tzu wrote, "He failed to realize that if he merely stepped into the shade, his shadow would vanish, if he sat down and stayed still, there would be no more footsteps."

I took many steps to outpace my shadows on the streets of London. And the footprints seemed to run in circles. Old thoughts swept me into old memories. What I thought was forgotten was remembered. It was the emotion, the turmoil and pain that shadowed me. A few conversations with Lydia surfaced. Isolated events left footprints here and there as I paced.

If Rachel had breast cancer, Australia was not an option. I had no insurance back in the U.S. and I of all people knew what it meant to not have insurance with a serious illness in the United States. The only thing I could think of was we would have to stay in England. We would have to get married by law so I could work there. Then there was the matter of work. What would I do?

My mind ran in circles, circles similar to the ones in Colorado after Lydia and I got the phone call from the blood bank. I had traveled the length of fourteen years and ran into the same footsteps with the same shadows.

I realized the more scenarios I built around what we might do the greater the fear. I was trying to protect myself emotionally and mentally by designing strategies yet it was having the opposite effect. My grief had thawed. The fear I thought was gone was simply frozen, lying in wait. Where at one point in my grief process I didn't care whether I lived or died, now, my slow return to life brought back my desire, my ability to care. Time had changed. I wanted more time. And my fear of losing Rachel returned me to the prison of time with a vengeance.

As I paced London I began to discern with greater clarity my fear's place of origin. Memory took me back into time, back to Lydia's words, her expressions, her eyes, mainly her eyes. I knew what it felt like to lose someone. I knew what was going to happen if Rachel was diagnosed with cancer. I knew. I knew. Fear told me that I knew.

The relationship between time and loss started to unfold. In the years since Monterey I watched with great pain the chasm between my grief's time and the clock the rest of the world kept. It was a phenomenon that I couldn't seem to reconcile.

I thought I was "getting over" the loss and coming back to life. It wasn't life I was coming back to; it was the harmonization of my time and the world around me that was coming back into sync.

I thought I had made it through the hard part. I had survived. I had found a reason to live. Loss's grip had lessened. I had returned to the present tense. Rachel and I were going to start a life in Australia. I would write. She would get her degree and we would go wherever that led. The darkness was over. The shadow of suicide that perpetually lingered no matter how fast I ran seemed to subside in the initial days with Rachel.

Again, I thought I had turned the corner when Rachel came into my life. And waiting for her test results made me question again whether there are any corners to turn.

I called Rachel in Bristol every night. She was calm. The power of past experience was my disadvantage. But since Rachel had never experienced something like this she was in her usual laid back mode. Intuitively she felt there was not going to be any cancer. One night as we spoke she said, "We'll just deal with it if it comes."

The grounding Rachel developed in her journey of Spirit was what grounded me during those days. Just the sound of her voice brought me to the present and she was right. I have dealt with whatever came.

She called me with the news. The lumps were benign. There was no relief in her voice. It was matter of fact. There was relief in mine.

But as I eased back into my equilibrium there still lingered the thought of where loss had taken me. The pacing of London's streets taught me the power of time and distance to move forward and grief's power to crumble both in a heartbeat. A length of time did not necessarily correlate with the distance from sorrow's epicenter to emotional safety. A single breath, one taxi ride, could bring it all tumbling down upon me. By its very nature my resiliency defined my fragility and my fragility defined my resiliency.

London warned me. No matter how far I go I still had to live with where I've been. And distance was an illusive illusion, just like time.

What Holds the Body, the Body Holds

Writing came easy for me. Unfortunately, publishing did not. Sandy, my agent in Sydney, did her best to get my first book in front of publishers in the U.S. It simply wasn't what they were looking for and a first-time fiction writer has to be extraordinary. Rejection after rejection piled up on my doorstep.

Still, I kept writing. I started another book. When Rachel and I spent the month on Phi Phi Island and I started writing the play, I had a remarkable shift.

Tess, one of the writers from Roland's classes was a Reiki master. She was in her fifties. The first time I saw her she had a shaved head, not uncommon for Buddhist nuns, but Tess's shaved head was for a cancer fundraiser back in Australia. Volunteers would gather donations of friends and family for cancer care and research by committing to shave their heads.

It was fairly apparent that Tess was not coming from a quiet, contemplative lifestyle of a Buddhist nun. Her demeanor was cast in exuberance. She absorbed life to its fullest and it exploded joyfully into everything she touched.

Tess offered us a Reiki blessing for our commitment ceremony. We accepted. Then she offered us individual Reiki sessions. Again, we accepted. I didn't know what I was getting into. My experience with bodywork was both sparse and sporadic. It mainly centered on medicinal massage. I still came from the mindset that the body was secondary to spirit. It was a transitory vessel to pass spirit from time into eternity. I had no idea the true nature of the body's role on this planet.

I lay fully clothed on the hotel bed. Tess didn't explain much, if anything. She just said relax and enjoy. She lightly placed her hands on various parts of my body. It felt pretty tame and basically pain free. But during the session there was one place where I experienced a pulsating pain – my right ankle.

When I was seventeen I broke my ankle playing basketball. The ankle cracked completely through when I landed wrong. I had a cast for six months. Of all the physically painful experiences I have encountered I was surprised that this minor event was where this tremendous amount of heat and hurt collected during the session. Outside of that the Reiki session was nothing spectacular. She said there might be some "stuff" coming up later. I thanked Tess and went for a swim.

The next day I woke up with several huge boils under each armpit. There was something releasing in my body. I was informed that boils were a possible sign of anger and their location under my armpits might indicate something hidden.

I had done a great deal of work on moving through anger, and there was much to move through. Any emotion that solidifies blocks the natural flow of life and anger's weight lay heaviest on my soul, and apparently lay dormant within my body.

Grief had a strong component of anger for me in the early years. And no matter how much I tried to maintain the fluidity of my anger and release it in the most appropriate way possible, there seemed to always be a residue left.

Still, the boils surprised me. Not only were they incredibly painful, it was a painful reminder of how much still remained of what I had thought was gone.

It was also my first experience with just how much the body collects. I began to witness a different relationship between my body and spirit. Somewhere within this physical frame was a critical key to the fluidity of life's movement, including my loss, especially my loss. The body held the keys.

It was not a shift in perspective that occurred instantaneously. But it was the beginning of my integration of body, emotion and spirit in a conscious way.

In the subsequent years I've encountered other bodywork specialists. I never seek them out. They just seemed to appear and see more in me than I do. I have encountered people who practice Zentherapy, acupuncture, the ancient Taoist technique of Chi Nei Tsang and a technique called Integrated Awareness. Each deals with blocked energy in the body.

I was in one session with Michael, a practitioner of Zentherapy. He was working on some innocuous part of my foot. When he gently pressed the top of my left foot a floodgate of emotion poured out of me. I literally sobbed. What kept coming up was the phrase, "I want my body back. I want my body back." I kept thinking of Matt and his emaciated body, Lydia's enormous pain, her shingles that crawled up her back and into her skull, and Bryan's incessant agonizing cries as he scratched my chest. I still carried the guilt of having a healthy body and in that guilt I had denied myself access to the physical part of my spirit. For the rest of the hour I simply wept. I wanted my body back.

When I made that commitment to search for where heaven and earth meet back in Monterey, I had no idea that it would lead me to the body. I started to see that heaven and earth could meet in the interchange between body and spirit. After the Reiki-induced boils had subsided, I experienced a flow of energy, a release. But the interesting part of that release was the unfolding of four stories I wanted to write; four books ascended to the surface. A surge of creativity was in full flight and I could see these books and the core of each took shape while Rachel and I were on Phi Phi Island.

Back in Sydney, I finished the second book. Sandy liked it. She started the rounds with that one and I started the third book.

I was also writing screenplays for full-length movies. She presented one screenplay to some production companies. A little nibble here and there kept me hopeful for a while.

In the meantime, Rachel had graduated with a Masters in Professional Writing. She then began integrating the various meditative and bodywork programs she had learned over the years into a unique process for helping people identify and access their passions and map them into an integrated whole. She worked with individuals and teams, assisting them in becoming aware of the subtle signals from within the body to rediscover their true passions and live life to the fullest. Her ability to create an environment for the client to truly explore their true essence was an ideal combination. We named the process Senssoma.

I worked with Rachel in looking deeper into the connection between the body and spirit and continued to write. I finished the third novel and two more screenplays, still no luck in publishing. My friends would ask how the writing was going. I'd say, "The writing's great. The publishing sucks, but the writing is great."

I love to write. The story woke me in the morning ready to play and we'd have such fun. It was like my woodpile at the age of three had become a keyboard and I'd ride the wind of words. But rejection after rejection wore me down.

The One That Doesn't Write

I was in San Francisco researching my fourth novel. Alan, my friend of so many years, and I were over in Berkeley. Alan had just bought me lunch, not for the first time. Alan was my Patron Saint of Pasta. Through the years Alan had fed me, given me a couch to sleep on and offered his car to me when I passed through San Francisco. It was common for Alan to clear the use of his car for me as soon as I landed. He knew I would want to go down to Half Moon Bay to sit amongst the memories, perhaps drop a petal or two into an ocean of ash.

We collected our salads and sat on the side of the curb on a busy street in Berkeley. I was eye level to a parked delivery truck's tailpipe. The setting of my latest book was to be partly in Berkeley and I was refamilarizing myself to the surroundings.

I was pretty discouraged about the lack of publishing. I was not even close to a potential sale.

I said to Alan, "I'm at the end of my money. I've given it all I have and nothing. I'm a complete failure, Alan. Nobody wants anything I've written. Maybe I should just give up."

Alan listened to my moaning with his usual compassion. Then he said, "The only unsuccessful writer is the one that doesn't write."

Alan just became my Patron Saint of Writing. Nothing could have meant more to me than Alan's words. I don't think a letter from a publisher could have rested deeper than his words of wisdom.

Writing was more to me than trying to make a living. The closer I examined why I needed to write the more the underlying motivations started to unearth. I needed to write to keep the fluidity of creativity alive within me. But I also needed to write, and be published, because if I could translate all the various experience I had encountered into stories, then maybe, just maybe, all of this would make sense. If I could publish, it would mean Lydia, Bryan and Matt's gift to me did not go wasted. I needed someone to share this common ground in the lonely journey of loss. I kept saying to Rachel after another rejection, "I just need to hear an echo."

I did not realize the extent of how the publishing was tied to the shifting of loss. There was a point where the meaninglessness of a loved one's death needed to shift into meaning. I have seen it manifest in other people in various ways. Some join support groups to help others. Others do volunteer work or raise funds for illnesses or issues related to the death of a beloved. I have also watched people deal with the apparent meaningless of tragedy and stay in such a state. Aside from giving meaning, there was another desire for my work to be published – money. I was at the end of the money. It was the endpoint of life in the pact I made when Matt died. I thought something would show up, some money would come, if I just did what I loved from a loving space.

I do not believe in doing work that brings harm, to others or to me. And I had spent enough time in jobs I didn't like, which I think is also quite harmful. Another pact I made with myself after Matt died was that I would not work just for money, or health insurance, ever again.

In the years I didn't have a car I felt that I would much rather walk to somewhere I want to go than to drive a nice, expensive car to some job I hate. Again, every lifestyle has its price.

In my darker moments I still couldn't shake the thought of ending my life. No matter how much the loss was shifting through my love for

Rachel, the bodywork, the writing, the meditations that wedded stillness and movement, there was always a trace of a solemn pact that I would not live someone else's life. I would rather die. The price of not writing was too high. Writing was the currency that fed my soul.

The Same Life

For many years the question of destiny had floated through my thoughts. In seminary they called it predestination. The discussion centered on what was free will and what was predestined, as if these were the only two options. In those days of youth it was more of an intellectual exercise for me to travel the various theologies through the centuries. But when Matt was born and he and Lydia almost died in childbirth, the question of whether it was destined or not became personal.

Who decided? Who was free?

In seminary the material presented on predestination was served with various points of view, all having an answer neatly packaged. I found it to be a large leap from the dusty precepts to the bedside of a parishioner's dying husband.

In the conservative context of Baptist theology I was supposed to have the answers for the ones I served. Even before Matt's birth and our own personal descent into chaos, I felt uneasy with answers that came tightly wrapped. The answer "I don't know" wasn't one of the options on the multiple-choice tests in seminary, nor was it comforting when sitting beside the dying.

In the crumbling of our lives many years before I still lived with wanting to know. Did all this happen for a reason? Did I do something? Did I not do something? Who is to blame?

There was no one to blame. Nobody did anything to us. One of the great lessons I have garnered in this journey is to not take life personally.

Nevertheless, the question of freedom and destiny was an undercurrent in everything I did, even up to the year 2003. I was blocked and didn't know why.

What I did not realize was how connected my stagnation was to grief. It was the age-old question "Why?" that riveted me to grief, as if the answer would free me and I could move on.

Any time I am in resistance I find myself in stagnation, in the same way that a fallen tree leads to a buildup of debris. I discovered that the question itself was part of the problem, not the solution. It was part of the debris that collected and it also kept my grief alive.

I had subconsciously used it to keep Lydia, Matt and Bryan alive. It was a Zen koan, a riddle that has no answer.

A friend once told me, "I can tell you my life and make it sound like the most horrible, painful life you've ever heard. I can tell you the same life and make it sound like the most beautiful, wonderful life you've ever heard. And it's the same life."

I discovered a freedom was on offer in each moment, embedded in the small seconds of every breath, layered in the body that carried me.

The large questions of life that weighed so heavily on me began to lift. I had been looking in the wrong direction. It was just a beginning, and quite often painful. Freedom is not all it's cracked up to be.

Freedom confronted me with what wasn't free within me. It was as if I was kneeling over a tiny creek dying of thirst. All I could scoop were tiny morsels while just on the other side of this thick forest was a rushing river teeming with life. I could hear the sound of the river through the trees. It drew me; I wanted to drink of the river, but for some reason I couldn't leave the creek. The small trickle of water was enough to keep me alive. I didn't know the distance, or the peril in the woods that may have awaited me if I ventured in the direction of the river. The day was coming, however, to either step into the forest towards the river, or die.

~ 283 ~

The Breath in Exhale

The cancer had started with three undetected spots on my mother's lungs. My father called with the news. He said they had decided not to do any chemotherapy. They spent their fifty-third anniversary in the hospital.

My mother never talked long on the phone. Even before the cancer she never said much about her physical pain and struggle in trying to walk again. Her cryptic responses were truthful and frank, but still cryptic. My father was the one that communicated to us about the progression of the disease.

Death neared. My father suggested I return to Georgia.

When I walked in the room, the boxes of medical supplies in the corner of the room brought back memories. I leaned over the bed and gently hugged her. The curved fingers of her arthritic hands cupped my cheeks. Her smile was spontaneous. Her words eased like a sigh.

I sat in the rocking chair next to the hospital bed in their bedroom. All the paraphernalia of the dying surrounded us – juice with a straw, lotion, and lip balm rested on a tray.

My mother had fought death all her life. It would be a mistake to think that all people shadowed by suicidal tendencies want to die. Her struggle with depression and suicide was a battle to live. It was her desperate desire for life that drew her in her frustration to the gate of death. And each time she found herself there at the border of life and death, she chose life, as painful as life was.

There were certain areas in our conversations that were off limits, certain times and places that we would never visit or revisit. Mother was not much for memory lane. We started on the surface. We spoke of her limited mobility, but how she could still get in a wheelchair for about an hour. We talked about how much she could or couldn't eat. We talked about talking.

Everybody dies differently. Lydia and I shared more than most. I don't believe it is possible to share all of oneself, but Lydia let me deep into her journey of dying. She was a very private person and I felt she made great efforts to show me herself so I could be there for Matt. Sitting next to my mother helped me realize the extent of Lydia's openness and just how difficult that was for Lydia to touch those places for me, and with me.

Matt and I entered his final days as we entered every day we had — open and in sync. I walked his pace and he let me as much or as little as he wanted to, but it was usually more than less.

But with Mother, I knew it was going to be a different journey.

Our time together in Georgia reflected much of the way we did life. I did not expect anything different. When I was leaving to go back to Sydney we spent our last minutes of the visit in cryptic conversation, both of us feeling this was to be our last.

Our hug goodbye looked like any of our other hugs. The words were like any other words we said when we parted company. We both stayed true to form, in character and in between beginning and endings.

We kept in touch by phone in the passing weeks, still in character and true to form.

Skip dropped everything in Dallas and went to help my father in Georgia. Hospice arranged overnight care. Both Skip and Dad said it was a matter of days.

My mother was quite upset when my father told her that Rachel and I were coming. She knew that we would only be coming for her funeral and she wasn't planning on dying anytime soon.

When we walked in the room I was surprised by how much she looked like Matt. Her hollow cheeks and weary sunken eyes pressed tight against the bone. Even her smile carried me into the memory of Matt and how he looked at this stage of his life.

She had come to the end. She was more open than the last time I was in Georgia. She shared some of her reflection over her seventy-two years. There was much she missed along the journey and she touched her lamentations with genuine openness and honesty. But she always stopped short of letting me into her deepest sorrows. After a time of silence I would ask her, "What are you thinking?"

Once her response was, "I'm thinking you're going to ask me what I'm thinking."

I never asked again.

Skip, Rachel and I had returned from town one night. Dad's shift was over. He was exhausted from the perpetual care and the imprint of preparatory grief. He went to sleep. Skip was going to take the night shift. Rachel and I went into the room for a moment to say goodnight. Since Mother was asleep we entered the room quietly and planned on leaving with a kiss on her forehead. I sat next to her, thinking it would be brief. Rachel took the chair on the other side.

In the stillness of the moment, I touched her hand and started to breathe in the rhythm of her breath. I slid my fingers under hers. The skin of her hand hung from the brittle bones.

Beneath the surface of each moment lies Moment, but there are some occasions where their interrelationship lifts into greater awareness. In the rhythm of the breath and the touch of the hand I found Moment touching us both. The fluidity of Spirit spread her in her sleep. It was a time when she was without resistance, which revealed the resistance itself. She had conversations with various departed friends and family. We only heard her responses.

She had a conversation with Luke, Lydia's father. She asked him where Matt and Lydia were. We don't know his answer, but apparently it sufficed for my mother. She said, "Oh, that makes sense."

There were presences in the room in those last days and I could feel their gentle flow of love for her. She battled hard to stay in this body that had begun shutting down. Many times she was close to death, but she returned, sometimes to consciousness, sometimes back to the rhythm of breath that weaves heaven and earth.

Someone telephoned to see how she was doing. Skip answered the call. He said, "Well, she's gone on to eternity. She's just decided to spend it here."

There was much for Mother to do in her last days. As I sat that night beside her, touching her hand, matching breaths, I thought of Bryan. Moment brought the memory of how I held him in the hopes that he would feel the pulsating love of God as his head rested on my pulsating chest.

She was asleep, shaping her spirit in a deeper layer, closer to where heaven and earth meet. I could feel the resistance in her body. Our spirits met within the breath.

Rachel sat next to us in silent support. I could feel the knots in Mother's spirit and how they reflected my knots. We traveled in a unique manner across the breath. My hand hovered about ten inches over the heat of her broken leg. She slept, deep in the dream, and we dreamed again Moment's dream.

Resistance is a survival mechanism. The fight to live, to survive, is innately part of the human condition. In many cultures death is described as the Destroyer.

As I sat next to my mother that night the unfolding of my own resistance surfaced. It was not a resistance to death that I experienced. It was the resistance to life, to the flow of life, to movement.

I once heard a friend say, "If nothing changes, nothing changes." At that time Matt and Lydia were still alive. I didn't want them to die, but their bodies had already turned on them. Their pain was daily. The resistance to change was what created my greatest pain, to want to keep them in that state would have been cruel, far more cruel than entering the change without resistance.

Rachel held a beautiful space for us as we sat with my mother for almost two hours. My hand drifted inches from the blockages in her spirit collecting, releasing and realigning heaven and earth. When it was finished, it was finished. Rachel and I said goodnight to her as she continued to dream.

Does the dream dream us or do we dream the dream?

On another night it was my shift to sleep the night in the single bed next to hers. Her frail features had started to mirror Matt's even more. The pattern of her breath and the anguish of her body echoed in my memory.

My sleep was restless. I kept waking up to see if she was still breathing. I kept thinking of the night Matt died and how I slept in his last hour. Ultimately I fell into a deep sleep. She coughed and it startled me into consciousness. I jerked my head off my pillow. In the delirium of not being fully awake or no longer asleep, I thought I was waking next to Matt on his last breath. I looked over expecting to see my son. Instead I looked at the frail body of my mother. Her breath was shallow, but steady, steadier than mine.

I thought I had reconciled with the hour I slept before Matt's death. On a conscious level, I had. Within the other layers of life, I had done much to rest in my peace. But in that state between suddenly waking from one dream into the other I was reminded of what I still carried and what I resisted in letting go.

I lay back on my pillow, one eye on the shadows lying on the ceiling and the other eye watching a pulsating heart just half a heartbeat out of sync. My spirit was wearier than my body. I was tired of the resistance. There had to be some way to break the barriers I had to letting go of this sorrow.

One Death Unfolds Them All

When my mother was healthy she usually woke around four in the morning. It was her favorite part of the day. She loved sitting on the enclosed porch as the sun started to light the mountain. In autumn it was even more spectacular to watch as some of the tree limbs, already leafless, spiraled into the bluing sky and other leaves still lingering on branches grew in color, frail in their waning days.

Now, in her last autumn days, I was staying in the house next to the one where she lay. It was Skip's banging on the door that stirred me in the early hours of morning's darkness.

He said she was close. She had been close before, many times before. But Skip said this looked closer. He said, "She may go soon, but she may last through the day. We don't know. But Dad and I agreed that you should know. Her breathing is changing."

I decided to take a quick shower and get ready for the day since it was not apparent her death was imminent. I was in the bedroom putting on my clothes when the gentle wind blew through me.

I knew the texture of that wind. And I knew she had just died. She passed by me, within me, and beyond me. She touched me with the breath of Spirit as it rode a gentle wind.

I relaxed my pace. It was finished.

When I left the house to go next door, another wind blew. This was a strong gale that pressed against my steps up the road to their house. It was autumn cold, a fresh clean cold that swirled like a dance around me. I knew that wind, too. It was the one that slammed against the window to wake me for Matt's last breaths. It was the one filled with power and strength. And I knew it was the collective wind that came to tell me of her goodbye.

My father was standing on one side of the bed, my brother on the other, when I entered the bedroom. Skip said she had just breathed her last a few moments before I entered.

In Matt's last days, I took lots of pictures. I needed to remember his last days because as we traveled through his physical deterioration I could not see it. I needed to look back unclouded by my love to see just how destroyed his body was. It helped my grief in the months and years ahead to see how he needed to die, to leave the gallows of his painful body and enter fully into the next dimension.

My eyes rested on my mother's breathless body. And I felt her spirit's breath on my face. I wanted to touch the warmth of her skin, just as I did Bryan's as his body emptied into winter. I wanted to sit next to her just as I did Lydia as I read the letter Lydia wrote to me, the words of remembrance and tender union. I wanted to see again where eternity meets between heaven and earth in spirit and body.

I wanted the impossible. I wanted those memories to be this memory. The death of one is as unique as the life of one. As much as memory tried to overlay other templates of sorrow onto the death of my mother, it was not to be.

I sat next to her body and spirit. I sat with her in the stillness of shared history. My memories were like a small rock descending softly to the bottom of clear pond.

I sat alone with my mother. Both Skip and our father needed time to assimilate their presence at her last breath. To be with another at the exact time timelessness sweeps through is a wonderful gift and it takes time to return to a temporal equilibrium. I did not experience this with my mother and so my vigil's reference point was of a different kind. We sat spread across time in the shared history, the common memory that was mother and child.

She birthed me. She watched me come into this world and now I was watching her leave.

I remembered her pulling my tooth as a child. I was in her lap in a rocking chair when she wrapped a string around the tooth that impeded the permanent one underneath. Her voice was comforting and calm as we rocked. She told me what was going to happen and why. I knew it was going to be painful, but it felt good to be resting against her chest and held safe by her gentle strokes of my hair and tender words. She counted to three. Some parents say they are going to count to three and then jerk the tooth out on two. But when my mother said she would pull at the count of three, I knew it would be on three.

I remembered the occasions when the pain was almost unbearable for her. She let me witness the difference between physical, emotional, mental and spiritual pain and how each has their own seasons and unique rhythm. She saw her inability to hide her seasons as a failing. I saw them as her greatest strength and my most treasured gift.

I sat next to her body letting memory flow into memory like turning a page on a photograph album. We shared what we could with the time allotted.

It was time to take her body away. And it was time for me to go back to the borrowed house and sit in the quiet. No more memories. Just the quiet that gifts a mountain morning in autumn.

It was good to be alone. I sat on the porch resting a cup of coffee on my leg and watching the morning sun move further from the silhouette of rolling mountains into the sky. I also watched as heaven moved further from earth. My unsettling began to emerge. My numbness thawed. Heaven left me once again in earth.

Rachel had to return to Sydney a few days before Mother died. On the phone she gently shed her tenderness over my withdrawal, giving me room to be whatever I needed to be. Skip, the one that probably knows me best, remained silently present. Like Mother, he never entered without an invitation, but his ability to lean a candle into my darkness was remarkably kind and insightful. Still, I was slipping into a prison of my own making.

My father and mother's house was empty. Skip was in the shower and I was waiting for him. We were about to go into town.

It was in the waiting for Skip and the reflection of what I was creating and couldn't stop that it happened. The wind that blew through me at her death had rested upon me again. In the briefest of moments, the loving presence of my mother's spirit passed by and left an invisible touch. No words, not even a thought, passed through me. Just the gentle breeze rested for an eternal second.

It was enough to dislodge me from the ethereal prison I had built. It was a beginning of a shift in me, an opening that still had far to go, but it was a beginning nonetheless. I was able to grieve and open to the world around me at the same time.

My father gave Rachel and me many of Mother's things, but the only thing that I truly wanted was a small mirror that sat facing her favorite chair in the living room. On the shelf she had a brass-plated round mirror encircled by the sun's rays. Between the rays of sun and the mirror were various stars and crescent moons. The value of the sun mirror was certainly not monetary. But to me, it was a symbol of where heaven and earth met that day; where the stars, crescent moons and sun met in the mirror's reflection. And where the wind set me free.

One Petal, One Kiss

On my way back to Sydney I had a couple of days' layover in San Francisco. Alan met me at the airport. I dropped him off at his office and proceeded south to Half Moon Bay. It was a beautiful morning, crisp and fresh. The sun settled nicely on the long stretch of white beach. For the first time in a long time I walked the curved bay's entire length. I picked up a long slim stick and walked nearer to the ocean, stopping a fair distance from the small lapping waves, just out of the reach of the morning tide. With the borrowed stick I carved four names instead of three – Bryan Caleb Allen, Lydia Ann Allen, Matthew Benjamin Allen and Wanda Ruth Allen. One name rested above the next, my mother's name sat closest to the ocean's edge.

These four names would last a day. When the sun set, the moon would take the names with the tide, back to from where they came.

It had been a long journey into death for my mother. I sat on the rocks at Half Moon Bay in a long journey of my own. I was still finding it difficult to let go deeply into the Is. The disturbance of my mother's death was reshaping my equilibrium again. Sitting on the beach, next to my ocean of ash, with names carved in sand waiting to disappear, I held a flower petal – one petal, one memory, one kiss.

It's Just a Dream

In a dream I opened a door and walked inside a room. The room was like a museum. Individual lights shone on rows and rows of exhibits encased in square glass on pedestals. Each exhibit held a piece of my life, not just any piece, though.

This room held all my hurt – encased in rows and rows of exhibition cases. I stood at the entrance. At the other end of the room was a door. I thought if I touched each one of these hurts maybe they would let me go. I thought my goal was to reach the door at the other end and move into a different chamber, another room, free from what was blocking me, holding me in pain. I desperately wanted to be free.

I walked past the first few exhibits to the center of the room. The first was at the time of my birth. The scene moved like a picture show as I was born by caesarean and whisked a hundred miles away to an intensive care. I watched the scene unfold in front of me. Another was looking into the mirror as a child, eyes blood red with tears. I watched the child watch the child. Another scene finished and I was on my way to the next. Hopefully closer to the door. As I slowly turned in a circle to survey the pieces of memory still left to touch that encased my hurt, I began to dissolve. My body became ash on the floor and my spirit started its descent into the chamber below. Slowly I was released into a deeper layer, healed of the hurt, into the chamber's chamber. The room that held me, held me no longer. And I awoke from the dream.

What had kept me together had kept me apart. Instead of being their ashes on my hands out at sea it was my hands on ash.

The body holds more gifts than I first realized. Through my attention and awareness of the subtle energies stored in the body I started another layer of the journey. The body has become like a library. My physicality does not stop on the edge of my fingers and toes that will ultimately succumb to ash. The universe, the physical dimensions of time and space, are not compartmentalized in separate beings.

There is something unique about our physicality, something precious; perhaps a clue into the wonderment of life lies within our bodies and this physical manifestation of Spirit. I had been afraid to embrace it because it was a collection of my hurts. To hold what is transitory was to experience the pain of loss. I had looked to transcend the body and its pain and misery, not to hold the body closer in awareness and intentionality.

Nothing in the universe is wasted. Spirit became flesh. What was the body to teach me? What gifts lay within skin and bones, the anatomy of Spirit? Somewhere in the interchange of heaven and earth I lived through Spirit, through illusion, in a body, within the dream.

I can see this dream as a horrible nightmare or a dream filled with beauty and love. I can embrace this dream as a blessing or a curse. Either way it is the same dream.

In the final analysis this is my dream. And what a wonderful dream it is. It is a dream beyond beginnings and endings, without a start or finish. It is the intricate dance of the physical, emotional and spiritual structures that unfold the mystery of me.

Matt was right. "The meaning of life is life itself."

As for me, I choose life, in all its shades and colors. I choose life. For in all of us is the capacity to live beyond the edge of ordinary... if we choose.

Epilogue

October 2008

Rachel and I went on vacation up to the Quinault, Washington. The seasonal rains had yet to begin and the sunlit beach glistened. The rhythm of the ocean sang in harmony with the soft breeze and waves encircled the huge boulders that have stood for centuries on their coastal watch.

Rachel was on the beach with some friends. I had wandered off to sit on one of the boulders. I watched the droplets fly into the air after crashing against the rock, and was reminded of my time in Mendocino. Once again I felt the familiar. The coastline had the look and feel of Mendo, the place I moved to after Matt died. It was along those Mendocino cliffs, next to this ocean, that I spent miles of moments gathering what was left, unfolding moments past and, unbeknownst to me, preparing for moments to come.

I tasted the sweetness of the Quinault on that October day and out of that sweetness I reflected on the pathways that brought me to that rock, that ocean's edge, that familiar place that nurtured me in my most fragile times.

I went further, to the memories that carried the collective of me. I went back to the first time I met Lydia when I was eleven. The first time I realized how much I loved her at the age of twenty when we sat that evening on the front lawn of her apartment laughing long into the night.

I returned to the time she told me she was pregnant with the child yet to be named, remembering both the sheer joy and absolute terror of becoming a father, and the self-questioning of what kind of father I would be.

I traced the silhouette of that night in the intensive care as Matt held my finger, both of us gripping each second begging for another one. The seconds came and went. For thirteen years seconds became minutes, rising like the waves swirling around the stone where I rested my bones that day in the Quinault.

I went through many memories of Lydia, Matt and Bryan and kissed each one with a deep sense of gratitude, just as I'd done for years with the Rose Ceremony. This time I didn't have the petals that touched my lips with each memory, but it was the same heart that each of their lives had touched and shaped in me.

After finding myself so utterly alone, I had traveled the world, and in my aloneness I found myself. In my unfolding I was in complete gratitude for what each of them had given me. Of all the many, many gifts, one of my most precious is second sight. I treasure most the lens of Spirit that I look through every day. I see clearly the transitory nature of life and how precious this collection of time within the landscape of timelessness is.

I bowed to this moment in gratitude for what I have been given and what I could give in return. Rachel had entered my life and I was given to love again. I have been honored to enter the lives of fellow sojourners where the phrase deep calls to deep reflects the blessing of their deepening of me.

I have been blessed.

On that sunny October day another memory passed through me. It was the day I spread the ashes of my children. It was the hours I spent at

Monterey Aquarium after I had dipped my ash-covered hands in the same ocean that I gazed upon.

As mentioned earlier, on that cold rainy day thirteen years earlier I sat waiting. For Matt and I had an arrangement. We had agreed that if he was okay he would send three dolphins to jump that day. I waited for hours, but no dolphins jumped. The cold and rain swept me further into my emptiness before night took me completely.

The memory of thirteen years earlier segued into this moment. I spoke to the Ancient One that was once my son. My thought formulated with a slight smile and a feeling of peace as I said to Matt, "You never did send those dolphins."

Just at that very moment three dolphins gently swam right in front of me. Three. Not four. Not two. Three. They didn't jump like I had envisioned they would thirteen years earlier. They simply sauntered by without a glance towards me. In my disbelief I shouted down to Rachel. I pointed to the dolphins. To my relief she acknowledged them. If they were an illusion then they were an illusion to us both. But they were not.

Loss and its healing elements are not linear. In this moment neither was time.

All those years ago I wanted so desperately to know Matt was okay. I wanted something, anything that would not only signal that he was still on journey, but that we were still on journey. I wanted to know the intertwining of our lives was still unfolding no matter the distance or dimension. That day in Monterey I just wanted a sign that he was okay.

As the dolphins passed me I realized the message was more than Matt was okay. I sat on the rock looking over the expanse with the most tender message I could have ever received. The message from Matt was not "I'm okay" but "You're okay."

As I walked in some distance from the others back to the car, with every step I looked for a small rock that was waiting for me. I carry a small triangular rock in my pocket. Some people think it is a gratitude rock, popularized in certain circles. Perhaps it is to some degree. But the deeper reminder to me when I caress this rock is this: everything is perfect just as it is. It is my Serenity rock. With every touch, this piece of earth says to me "everything is okay."

Truly, in this moment, everything is okay, perfect in its unfolding.

About the Author

Several years ago Benjamin appeared extensively in the media beginning with the *New York Times, Dateline, The Today Show, Good Morning America, 20/20* and various local newspapers, especially *The Dallas Morning News*. His story also featured on *The Oprah Winfrey Show*. The subject matter focused on the tragic circumstances his family endured.

Lydia, his wife, received a blood transfusion with HIV during the birth of their first child, Matt. He and Lydia had another child, Bryan, before they were informed of her infection. Consequently, his wife and their two children died, the first being in 1985 and the last death was in 1995.

In the midst of all this, one TV producer approached him to secure the rights to make a film about his life. He declined. Many people asked him to write his story, knowing how much it could potentially help others. He was not ready.

Finally, after many years of emotional and spiritual exploration, he came to a place of peace. This book, *Out of The Ashes: Healing in the Afterloss*, details that journey. Portraying normal people in abnormal circumstances, the book shows how he, and those he loved and lost, came to a deeper connection with life in the embrace of death.

It is an examination of what loss can take, but what it can also give. It is not a book about HIV/AIDS. It is a book that offers practical tips for dealing with any type of loss and moving into acceptance and healing.

Benjamin has worked with grieving individuals and groups for decades. He has also been trained and certified by The Grief Recovery® Institute (GRI). Benjamin began his career as a Southern Baptist minister and was the pastor of Pacifica Baptist Church in California. He worked for the Christian Life Commission of the Baptist General Convention of Texas from 1985-1991. He was the founding Director of the Dallas AIDS Interfaith Network, and a member of the Texas Legislative Task Force on AIDS and the National AIDS Commission. From 1991-1995 he worked with the HIV Research Group at the University of Texas Southwestern Medical School in Dallas, Texas. Southwestern Medical School in Dallas, Texas.

His journey has brought him to a place of peace. As with everyone, Benjamin is still on the journey of healing. Once asked what he now believes, Benjamin responded, "I have no labels, no attachment to a particular belief. All I know is that I am a human, born of Spirit. And in Spirit, there is only love."

He now lives at Lake Tahoe, Nevada where he writes and delivers personal growth programs.

Thank You

Out of the Ashes: Healing in the Afterloss chronicles my journey — a world of pain and grief following unspeakable loss. When you are in the depths of pain, you feel like the pain will last forever, that it will never go away. But I am here to tell you that it is possible to come to a place of healing and peace. You can even find a new ways to connect with meaning and purpose with the one you lost.

I share my story so you will know you are not alone. My mission with this book is to encourage you and give you hope. Please give yourself permission to lean into your loss, whether it be fresh or ancient history. Everyone experiences loss. It is my hope that as I share how I made it through the Afterloss of sorrow into healing, you will see how the losses in your life can discover healing, too.

There is more to our journey together if you wish. Please visit TheAfterLoss.com where I blog regularly about the healing process. You can sign up there to receive more information and valuable resources. Join our active Facebook community at Facebook.com/theafterloss.

Also watch for my forthcoming publication *Living in the AfterLoss Guidebook*. This companion to *Out of the Ashes: Healing in the Afterloss* will provide you a deeper place of reflection and an awareness of your own healing journey.

You do not need to explore this new world of the Afterloss alone.

In this Guidebook you will discover:

- The important elements in the healing journey.

- How to embrace preparatory grief so you are able to start the healing process.

- How to live in The AfterLoss – the way to move through grief into a more meaningful, whole experience of life.

- How to honor the one you have lost, and shift the pain into an experience of peace and acceptance.

Made in the USA
Monee, IL
05 June 2022